Textbook of Removable Partial Prosthodontics

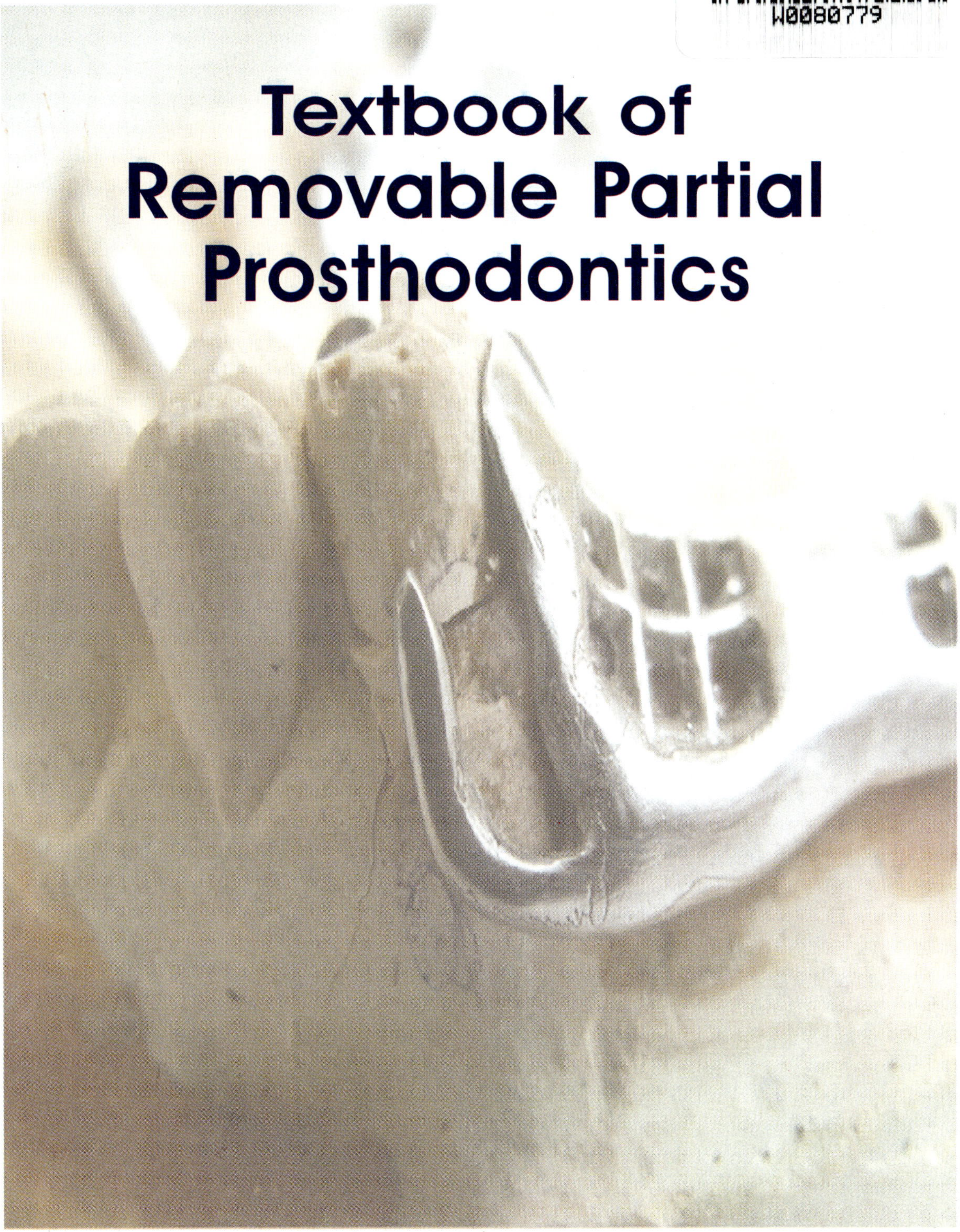

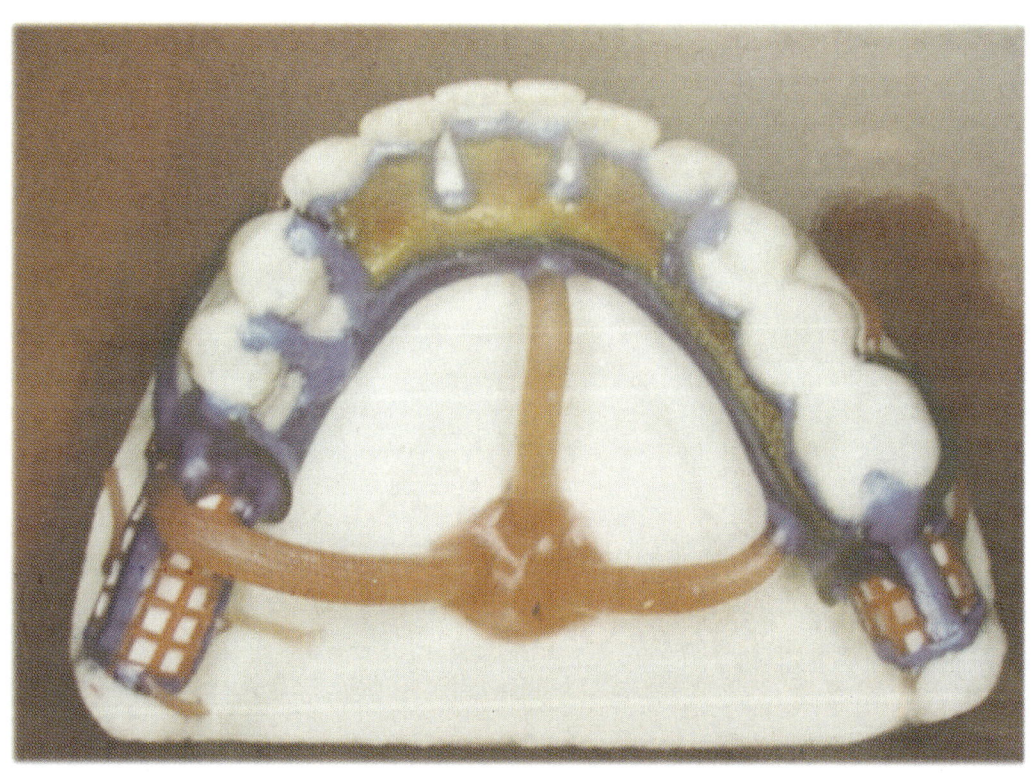

Textbook of Removable Partial Prosthodontics

Sharad Gupta
MDS (GDC & H, Mumbai)

Associate Professor
Department of Prosthodontics
Institute of Dental Studies and Technologies
Modinagar, UP

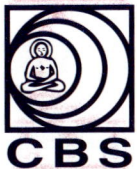

CBS

CBS PUBLISHERS & DISTRIBUTORS

New Delhi • Bangalore • Pune (India)

Textbook of
Removable Partial
Prosthodontics

ISBN : 978-81-239-1721-4

First Edition : 2009

Published by Satish Kumar Jain and produced by Vinod K. Jain for
CBS Publishers & Distributors
4819/XI, Prahlad Street, 24 Ansari Road, Daryaganj, New Delhi 110 002 (India)
Fax: 011-23243014 • e-mail: cbspubs@vsnl.com; delhi@cbspd.com
Website: www.cbspd.com

Branch Offices:

Bangalore: Seema House 2975, 17th Cross, K.R. Road, Banasankari 2nd Stage, Bangalore 560070
Fax: 080-26771680 • e-mail: cbsbng@gmail.com

Pune: Shaan Brahmha Complex, Basement, Appa Balwant Chowk, Budhwar Peth, next to Ratan Talkies, Pune 411002
Fax: 020-24464059 • e-mail: pune@cbspd.com

Printed at:
Swastik Packaging, Patparganj, Delhi-92

to

my parents
who taught me
'qualification is the biggest asset'

my lovely wife Vishakha
who continues
to reform me from 'good to great'

my son Soham
who is
the joy of my life

my teachers, patients and students

Foreword

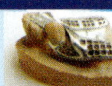

It gives me immense pleasure to write the Foreword to *Textbook of Removable Partial Prosthodontics* written by one of our students Dr Sharad Gupta. He has done his thesis on cast partial dentures. During the course of his research he has gone into the depth of the subject, which has enamored him to come out with a book on removable partial dentures for students and dentists.

The art and science of partial dentures prosthodontics may be complex and challenging. The understanding of the subject with its variations remains ambiguous. Success in partial denture treatment is dependent on the adherence to a number of inescapable principles. This book will provide information on commonly used terminologies, components of partial dentures with illustrations, the biomechanical principles for designing, details in surveying, examination, diagnosis and treatment planning, support of the tissues and the occlusal considerations.

The book also caters to the laboratory procedures for fabrication of the cast removable partial denture. This book would provide a pragmatic approach to the partial denture designing, making the daunting task simple, interesting and easy. This can be read by both students and dentists alike for solutions when treating patients of removable partial dentures.

I wish this book a success and recommend its reading by practising dentists.

Dr Sabita M. Ram

Professor and Head
Department of Prosthodontics
D.Y. Patil Dental College and Hospital
Navi Mumbai

Acknowledgements

No work is a man's work alone. Great thinking experience and above all destiny intermingles to bring into existence what was once just a thought.

I express my first gratitude to my profession which inspired me to become a better student and transformed me into a teacher and clinician. I extend my thanks to all my teachers, my students and my patients from whom I learned and continue to learn.

I would like to sincerely appreciate late Mr. B R Sharma for his motivation and belief in my work. Special thanks to Anant Sharma for his association with this work .

My gratitude to the publishers and their entire team working on this project under the dynamic and experienced guidance of Mr. Y N Arna, Editor-Director, CBS.

Sharad Gupta

Preface

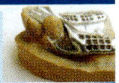

Removable partial prosthodontics is one of the major branches of prosthodontics. Majority of the patients seeking tooth treatment are primarily partially edentulous. In this era of dental advancement and innovations, newer modalities like fixed partial denture and more recently titanium implants have been the front-runner for replacement of missing teeth.

Over and above 65,000 possible combinations of partially edentulous situations can exists. Even the modern treatment approach with dental implants and fixed partial denture offers no panacea for all the situations. Treating our patients with only one approach can lead to disaster in waiting. The science of conventional removable partial prosthodontics has stood the test of time. It comes to rescue for a vast variety of partially edentulous patients not amenable to any other treatment modality. The main aim behind any restorative work should be to restore back our patients to optimum function, aesthetics and comfort. It is also important to take into consideration the biomechanics of partially edentulous arches and the socioeconomic factors.

Removable partial prosthodontics encompasses a wide range of solutions for difficult dental situations. Provision of precision attachments, stress breakers along with advancements in laboratory materials and techniques renders almost any situation restorable to original.

My motivation for writing this textbook was both small and big. It was my dream and my understanding that there was a need for creating a work which would catalyse an average clinician into a successful removable partial denture practitioner. With almost 80% of partial dentures being designed by the laboratory technicians, fabrication of partial denture is done more by guess-work and personal preference for the design.

Any reader of this text will benefit from an in-depth understanding and preciseness of thoughts on almost all aspects of the subject. The entire text is discussed in 8 chapters. Each chapter is conceptually framed and to the point to nearly 'spoon-feed' the reader.

I would like to advise the reader that this text would be better understood and of great use after one has gone through standard textbooks on the subject like those by MacCracken & Steward. Students appearing for dental postgraduate examinations will benefit the most by the original multiple choice questions given at the end of every chapter.

To conclude, I have put in all my clinical and laboratory knowledge gained over the years on the subject for your reading. I believe my best work on the subject is still to come for I live by the words of 'Miguel De Unamuno'

"To achieve the impossible
one must think the absurd;
to look where everyone else has looked,
but to see what no one else has seen".

Sharad Gupta

Contents

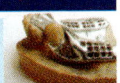

Foreword by Sabita M. Ram   vii

Preface   ix

1. Introduction, Terminology and Classification of Partially Edentulous Arches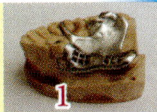

2. Component Parts of Removable Partial Denture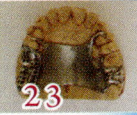

3. Biomechanics and Principles of Designing Removable Partial Denture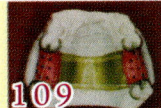

4. Surveying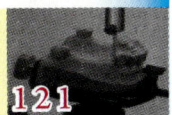

5. Examination, Diagnosis, Treatment Planning, Mouth and Abutment Preparation for Removable Partial Denture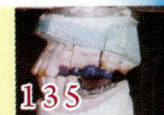

6. Support and Impression Procedures for Removable Partial Denture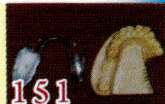

7. Laboratory Procedures in Fabrication of Removable Partial Denture Framework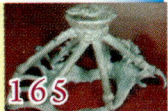

8. Planning Occlusal Relationship for Removable Partial Denture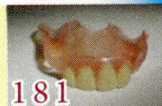

Suggested Reading   187

References   189

Index   191

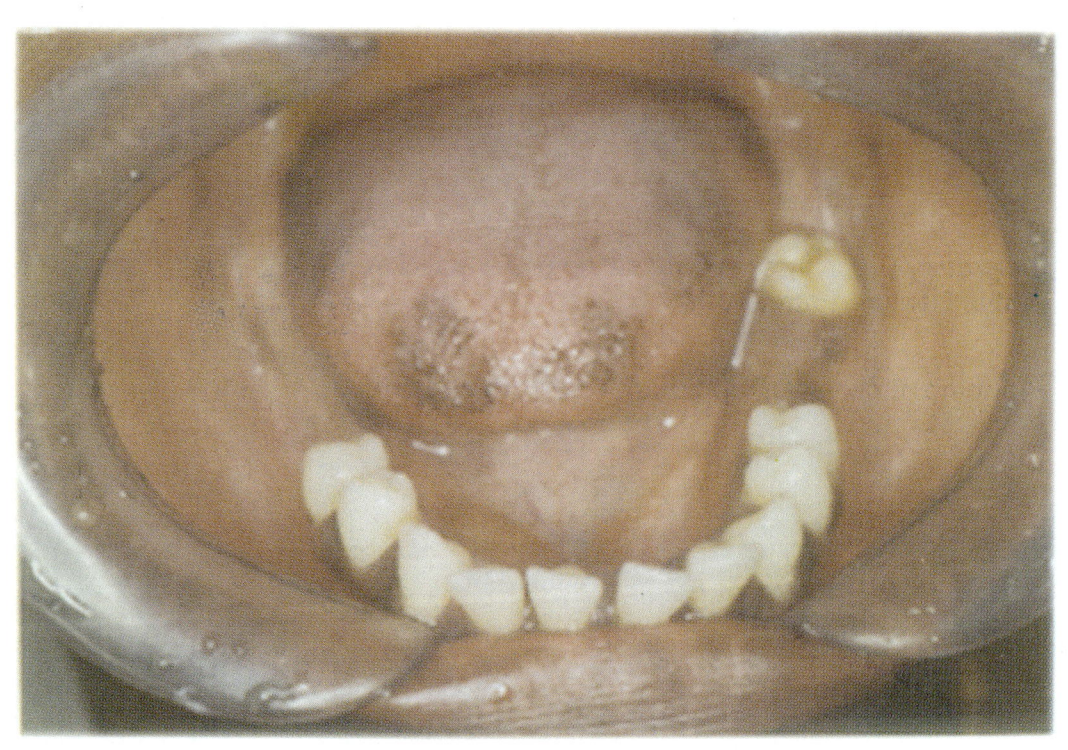

Introduction, Terminology and Classification of Partially Edentulous Arches

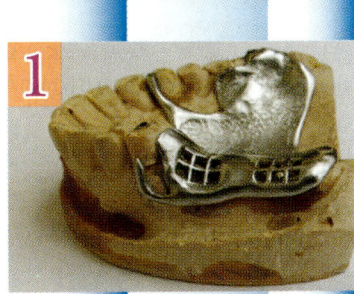

- ❑ The partially edentulous state
- ❑ Pattern of tooth loss and effects of partial edentulism
- ❑ Prosthesis selection for partially edentulous patients
- ❑ Rationale for removable partial dentures
- ❑ Component parts of cast partial denture
- ❑ Classification of partially edentulous arches
- ❑ Terminology related to cast partial dentures

THE PARTIALLY EDENTULOUS STATE

The loss of teeth most often occurs as a result of failure to maintain oral hygiene and plaque control measures. Poor oral habits leads to destruction of periodontium and tooth mobility ensues. Parafunctional habits may further exacerbate the situation causing irreversible damage and finally loss of tooth, leading to a state of partial edentulism (Fig. 1.1).

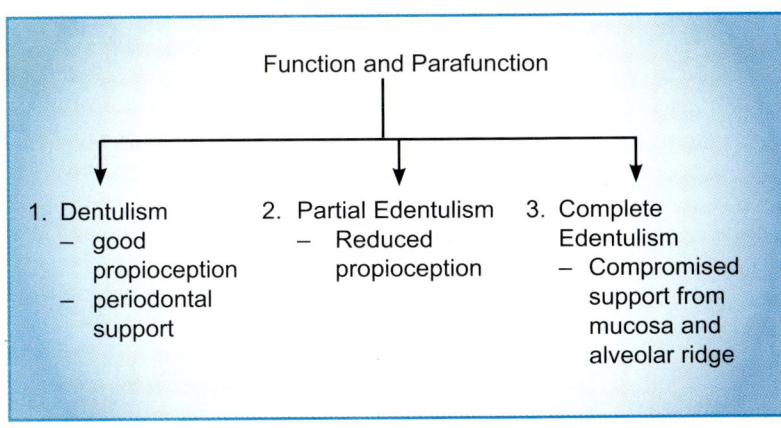

Function and Parafunction

1. Dentulism
   - good propioception
   - periodontal support

2. Partial Edentulism
   - Reduced propioception

3. Complete Edentulism
   - Compromised support from mucosa and alveolar ridge

Fig. 1.1: Integrity of masticatory system is challenged with loss of teeth

PATTERN OF TOOTH LOSS AND EFFECTS OF PARTIAL EDENTULISM

According to **Brewer (1980),** loss of patient's natural dentition follows following pattern:

Maxillary posteriors > Maxillary anteriors > Mandibular posteriors > Mandibular anteriors.

Mandibular canines are frequently the last remaining tooth in the mouth.

The consequences of partial loss of natural dentition are numerous and varied. Following are some important consequences.

1. Esthetic alterations.
2. Tipping, migration, rotation of remaining dentition.
3. Extrusion of opposing teeth in the endentulous space.
4. Loss of facial support.
5. Mandibular deviation.
6. Reduced vertical dimension with loss of posterior teeths.
7. Shortening of morphogenic face height and overclosure.
8. TMJ dysfunction.
9. Loss of alveolar bone and residual ridge resorption.
10. Loss of mastication.
11. Altered speech.

Selection of Prosthesis Type for Partially Edentulous Patients

Whenever possible a partially edentulous situation should be best restored with Fixed partial dentures or dental implants. Fixed partial dentures are better tolerated by patients and provides better health and function. However, there are situations which are non-restorable with fixed partial prosthesis and are best served with removable partial dentures.

INDICATIONS FOR REMOVABLE PARTIAL DENTURE

1. The Distal Extension Situation

When there are no teeth, posterior to the edentulous space, it could be a unilateral or a bilateral situation. Removable partial dentures are the best means of rehabilitating distal extension situations especially when placement of implants is also not feasible. Removable partial dentures also provides vertical support from the residual ridge in distal extension situation.

2. Long Edentulous Span

Removable partial dentures will provide dual support both from the residual ridge and from the teeth on the opposite side of the arch. Also, abutment teeth on the edentulous side are not jeopardized to horizontal or torquing stresses generated by the Flexion of a long span bridge.

3. Cross Arch Stabilization and Bracing

Rigidity of removable partial denture components and careful designing stabilizes the prosthesis against mediolateral and anteroposterior forces. Periodontally weakened teeth are thus splinted by cross arch effect.

4. Recent Extractions

Tissue changes are inevitable following extractions. An all acrylic temporary removable partial denture is the best replacement.

5. Esthetics

Greater esthetics in the anterior region are better established with a removable partial denture especially when there is both soft and hard tissue loss and patient is not willing for augmentative and regenerative therapy.

6. Transitional Prosthesis

For systemically ill or for psychological reasons, removable partial dentures enables an individual to make the transition to complete edentulism with minimum psychic trauma.

7. Abnormal Maxillomandibular Relationships

Patients with arch size, shape and position discrepancies are better restored with removable prosthesis.

8. Alterations of Vertical Dimension

Removable prosthesis (overlay, splint) can be used for determining the exact amount of vertical opening that a patient requires when increase in the vertical dimension of occlusion is contemplated as a part of overall treatment.

9. Restoration of Intraoral Maxillofacial Defects

Removable prosthesis like obturators and velum are successfully used for restoring acquired and congenital intraoral defects.

10. Patient's Desire for More Conservative and Economical Procedure

Sometimes due to economic constraints and unwillingness of patient for irreversible procedures like tooth structure removal for receiving fixed partial dentures, removable partial dentures can be fabricated when otherwise a fixed prosthesis could have served better.

RATIONALE FOR REMOVABLE PARTIAL DENTURE SERVICE

Age of an individual is found to be directly related to the tooth loss. The greatest incidence of partial edentulism is reported in the 35 to 54 year old age group. Molars are the most common teeth lost resulting in overall higher incidence of distal extension situations.

Dental implants can be successfully used for restoring partial edentulous cases including distal extension free end saddles. However, not all patients are candidates for dental implant therapy. Main contraindications for dental implant includes patients with uncontrolled systemic conditions, high dose radiations, smokers, and those with compromised bone types. Conventional fixed partial dentures, may also be ruled out for replacement of teeth in partially edentulous situations due to factors like age of the patient, weak abutment, excessive length of span, poor oral hygiene and lack of oral hygiene motivation.

Removable partial dentures when properly designed and fabricated can prove to be a definitive treatment modality for partially edentulous situations not amenable to restoration by any other means.

COMPONENT PARTS OF A CAST PARTIAL DENTURE

A removable partial denture is a prosthodontic restoration that supplies teeth and associated structure to a partially edentulous arch and that can be removed and inserted by the patient (Fig. 1.2).

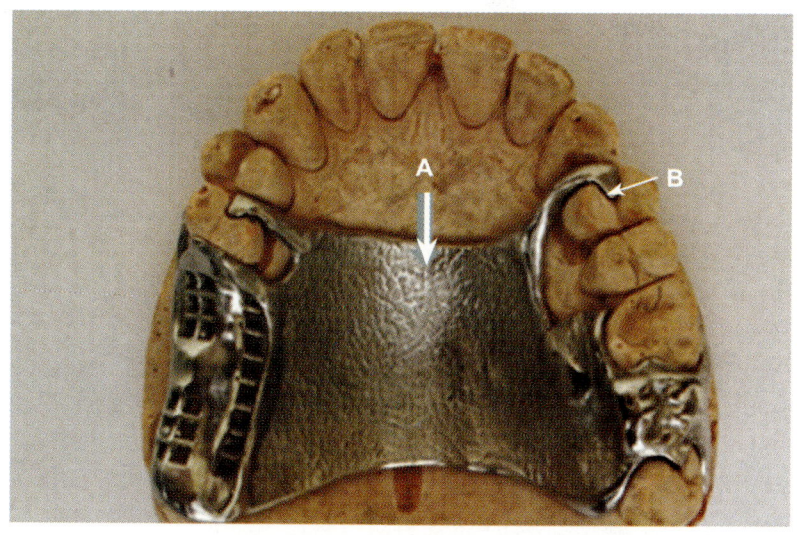

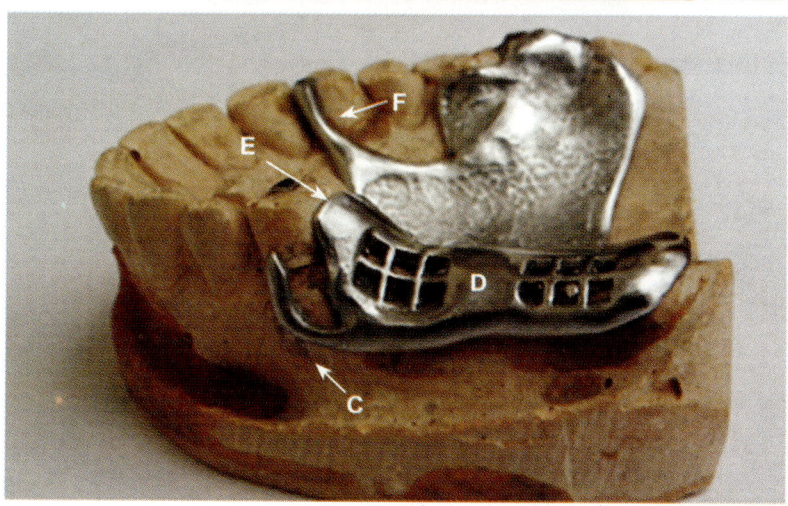

Fig. 1.2: Component parts of cast partial denture framework: (A) Major Connector, (B) Rest, (C) Direct Retainer, (D) Minor Connector, (E) Proximal Plate, (F) Indirect Retainer

TYPES OF REMOVABLE PARTIAL DENTURES

1. According to fixation to the natural Dentition.
   a. **Extracoronal:** retention by engaging tooth undercuts by clasps which are part of prosthesis.
   b. **Intracoronal:** Part of Retentive unit is placed within the confines of a restored natural tooth.
2. According to the support
   a. **Tooth borne:** When the removable partial denture is supported anteriorly and posteriorly by abutment teeth.

    b. **Tooth tissue borne:** When support for removable partial denture is obtained both from the remaining natural teeth and associated residual alveolar ridge.

3. According to the Material used
    a. **Metallic:** e.g. gold alloys, base metal alloys (cobalt-chromium), titanium alloys.
    b. **All acrylic:** e.g. cross-linked heat cure acrylic resin (methyl methacrylate)
    c. **Flexible partial dentures:** e.g. monomer free acetal resin (Dental D, Valplast).

OBJECTIVES OF REMOVABLE PARTIAL DENTURE

1. Preservation of teeth and tissue that will enhance the removable partial denture design and promote oral health.
2. To enhance masticatory function.
3. To distribute the occlusal load equally between the teeth and associated alveolar ridge.
4. To improve esthetics, phonetics and comfort besides overall health, general and psychosocial well being of the patient.

CLASSIFICATION OF PARTIALLY EDENTULOUS ARCHES

The primary purpose for creating a classification system for partially edentulous arches is to enable the dentist to clearly communicate to a listener or reader the condition of an oral cavity in which missing teeth are to be replaced with a prosthesis. Also, a workable classification system, aid in the learning of the fundamentals of design of cast partial denture. **There are around twelve and more classification system taught and followed worldwide for some 65, 534 possible partially edentulous situations** (Table 1.1).

Kennedy's Classification (Figs 1.3A to D)

According to Miller (1970), in a survey of American dental schools it was found that Kennedy Classification was most commonly followed. It was found to be simple, logical and workable, classification system.

    Kennedy (1925) divided all partially edentulous arches into four classes according to the frequency of occurrence.

	Table 1.1: Various classification systems for partially edentulous arches	
	Classification system	*Sailent features*
1	Cummers (1920)	• First recognized system. Based upon number and position of direct retainers classified arches from class I through class IV.
2	Kennedy's (1925) * (described in detail later in the chapter)	• Based on the relationship of the edentulous spaces to the abutment teeth. • Most widely and commonly followed. • It also forms the basis of two more classification namely: Applegate Kennedy and Swenson.
3	Bailyn's	• Classified saddles on the basis of tooth borne, tissue borne or a combination of both.
4	Neurohr's	• Complex classification (its of little use.)

5	Mauk's	• Classified on the basis of
		  i. Number, length and position of the spaces.
		  ii. Number and position of the remaining teeth.

6	Godfrey's	• Based on the location and extent of the edentulous spaces, e.g. anterior 4 tooth space or a posterior space.
7	Beckett's	• Class 1: Tooth borne saddle Class 2: Mucosa borne saddle Class 3: Inadequate abutments to support the saddle and inadequate mucosa support.
8	Friedman	• Based on the boundaries of the spaces. A: An anterior tooth bounded space. B: A bounded posterior space C: Posterior free end/cantilever situation
9	Austin ledge	• Not widely used A: Anterior space B: Posterior space Bi: Bilateral missing teeth X: Free end denture base
10	Skinner's	• Based upon the relationship of the abutment teeth to the supporting residual alveolar ridge.
11	Applegate-Kennedy's	• Modification of Kennedy system • Based upon the ability of the abutment teeth bounding the edentulous space to provide support. • Class I to Class IV are similar to Kennedy's classification. • Class V: An edentulous situation in which teeth bound the edentulous space anteriorly and posteriorly but where the anterior tooth is not suitable for support. • Class VI: An edentulous situation in which the boundary teeth are capable of providing total support to the prosthesis.
12	Swenson's	• Same as Kennedy but with slight modification. Kennedy's Class I is Swensons Class II and vice versa.

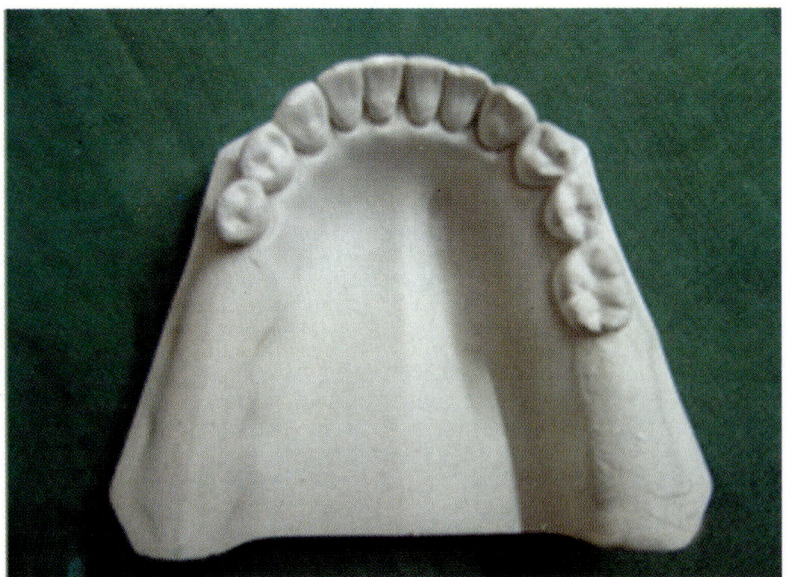

Fig. 1.3A: Class I (72%)

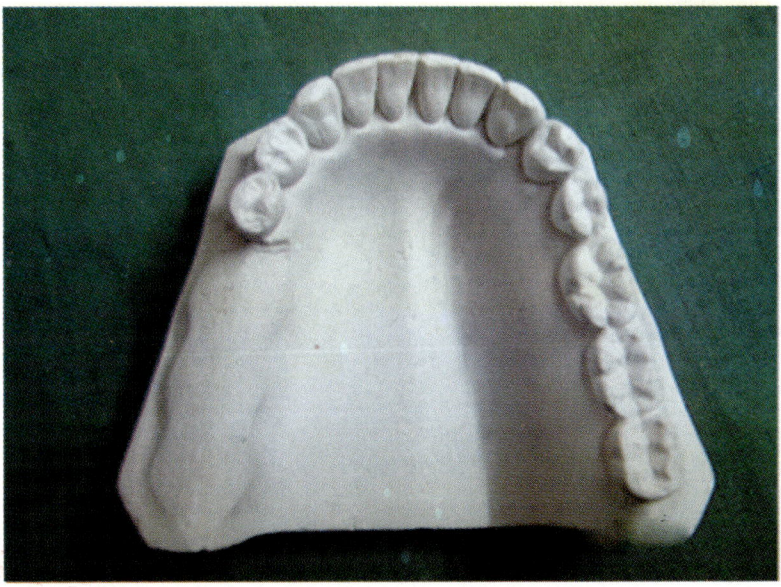

Fig. 1.3B: Class II (14%)

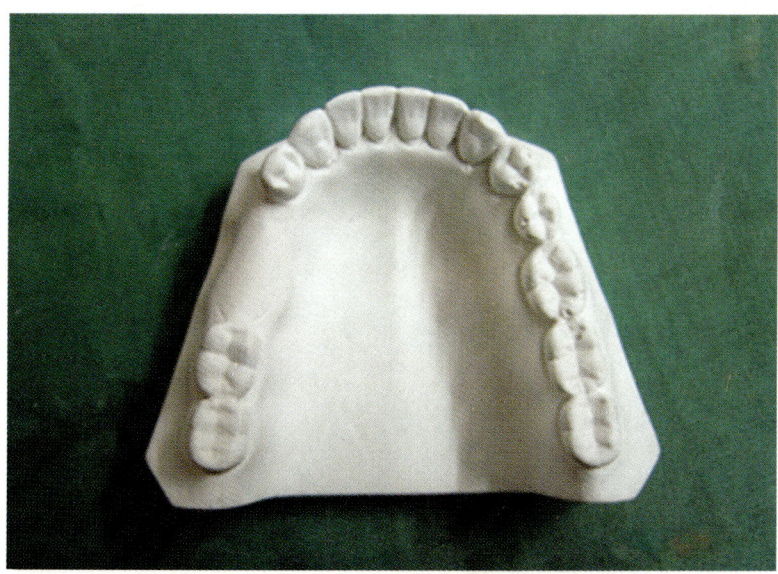

Fig. 1.3C: Class III (8.5%)

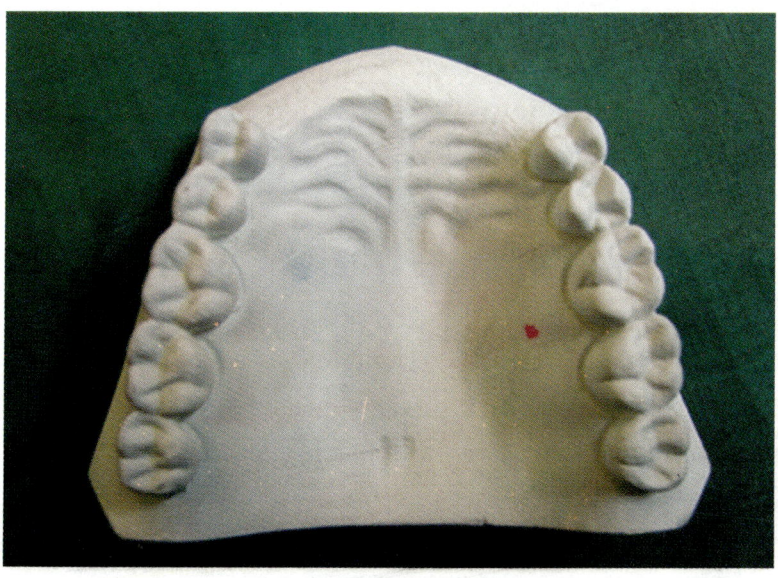

Fig. 1.3D: Class IV (3%)

Figs 1.3A to D: Kennedy's classification of Partially edentulous arches

Class I (72%)*   : A partially edentulous arch in which there are bilateral edentulous areas present posterior to the remaining natural teeth.

Class II (14%)* : A partially edentulous arch in which a unilateral edentulous area is located posterior to the remaining natural teeth.

Class III (8.5%)*: A partially edentulous arch in which there is a unilateral edentulous area with natural teeth remaining both anterior and posterior to it.

Class IV (3%)*   : A partially edentulous arch in which a single edentulous area, is located anterior to the remaining natural teeth and it crosses the midline.

* Incidence of occurrence

Applegate Rules Governing Kennedy's Classification (Table 1.2)

Following eight rules given by Applegate (1954) governs application of Kennedy's classification to any partially edentulous situation.

Table 1.2: Applegate rules	
Rule 1	Classification should follow mouth preparation since further extractions would alter it.
Rule 2	If the third molar is missing and not to be replaced it is not considered.
Rule 3	Third molars if present and are to be used as abutments. They are considered in determining the classification.
Rule 4	If a second molar is missing and is not to be replaced it is not considered in the classification.
Rule 5	The most posterior edentulous area determines the classification.
Rule 6	Edentulous area other than those determining the classification are termed as modifications and designated by their numbers
Rule 7	The extent of modification area have no bearing. It is the number of such areas that is the determining factor.
Rule 8	Class IV have no modification area possible.

Sequence of Partial Denture Treatment		
STEP 1	**Patient education**	Information regarding benefits of removable partial denture, types of removable partial denture material available, limitations of removable partial denture service. Proper knowledge regarding handling of prosthesis, oral care and maintenance of prosthesis should be provided.
STEP 2	**Diagnosis, treatment planning, prognosis, design consideration and mouth preparation**	Clinical and radiographic examination should be done. Correction of hard and soft tissue pathology. Use of dental surveyor to facilitate the design of removable partial denture.
STEP 3	**Establishing support for distal extension denture base**	Special corrected impression techniques and fabrication of altered cast. Functional impression for broad coverage of residual ridge.
STEP 4	**Establishment and verification of occlusal relations and tooth arrangements**	Jaw relations are made after verifying the fit of denture framework. Opposing occlusion is also verified and corrected for interference and deviation.
STEP 5	**Initial placement procedure**	Processing errors are corrected and processed bases perfected to the basal seat.Functional reline of denture bases are done at this stage for distal extension situation, if altered cast was not fabricated earlier.
STEP 6	**Periodic recall**	4–6 months periodic recall is essential. The relationship of framework to the abutments and the fit of denture base to supporting tissue should be checked.

TERMINOLOGY

The terminology given here is adopted from Glossary of Prosthodontic Terms (GPT 8) and includes most commonly used terms in cast partial denture prosthodontics. Terminology is given alphabetically.

1. Altered Cast

A final cast that is revised in part before processing a denture base called also corrected cast, modified cast.

2. Altered Cast Partial Denture Impression

A negative likeness of a portion or portions of the edentulous denture bearing area(s) made independent of and after the initial impression of the natural teeth. This technique employs an impression tray(s) attached to the removable dental prosthesis framework or its likeness.

3. Andrews Bridge

The combination of a fixed dental prosthesis incorporating a bar with a removable dental prosthesis that replaces teeth with the bar area, usually used for edentulous anterior spaces. The vertical walls of the bar may provide retention for the removable component. First attributed to James Andrews.

4. Angle of Gingival Convergence

According to Schneider, the angle of gingival convergence is located apical to the height of contour on the abutment tooth. It can be identified by viewing the angle formed by the tooth surfaces gingival to the survey line and the analyzing rod or undercut gauge in a surveyor as it contacts the height of contour.

5. Clasp Assembly

The part of a removable dental prosthesis that acts as a direct retainer and/or stabilizer for a prosthesis by partially encompassing or contacting an abutment tooth. Components of the clasp assembly includes the clasp, the reciprocal arm, the cingulum, incisal or occlusal rest, and the minor connector.

6. Combination Clasp

A circumferential retainer for a removable dental prosthesis that has a cast reciprocal arm and a wrought wire retentive arm.

7. Combination Syndrome

The characteristic features that occur when an edentulous maxilla is opposed by natural mandibular anterior teeth including loss of bone from the anterior portion of the maxillary ridge. Overgrowth of the tuberosities, papillary hyperplasia of the hard palate's mucosa, extrusion of lower anterior teeth, and loss of alveolar bone and ridge height beneath mandibular removable dental prosthesis bases. Also called anterior hyperfunction syndrome.

8. Continuous Bar Connector

A metal bar usually resting on the lingual surfaces of mandibular anterior teeth to aid in their stabilization and act as an indirect retainer in extension base partial removable dental prostheses.

9. Continuous Clasp

In removable dental prosthodontics, a circumferential retainer (clasp) whose body emanates from an occlusal rest and extends across the buccal or lingual surfaces of more than one teeth before engaging an undercut on the proximal wall farthest from the occlusal rest.

10. Continuous Gum Denture

An artificial denture consisting of porcelain teeth and tinted porcelain denture base material fused to a platinum base.

11. Extension Based Partial Removable Dental Prosthesis

A removable prosthesis that is supported and retained by natural teeth only at one end of the denture base segment and in which a portion of the functional load is carried by the residual ridge.

12. Fulcrum Line

An imaginary line, connecting occlusal rests, around which a partial removable dental prosthesis tend to rotate under masticatory forces. The determinants for the fulcrum line are usually the cross arch occlusal rests located adjacent to the tissue borne components.

13. Gillett Bridge

Eponym for a partial removable dental prosthesis utilizing a Gillet clasp system, which was composed of an occlusal rest notched deeply into the occlusal axial surface with a gingivally placed groove and a circumferential clasp for retention. The occlusal rest was custom made in a cast restoration.

14. Milling

The machining of proximal boxes recesses, or other forms on cast restorations to be used as retainers for fixed or removable prostheses.

15. MORA Device

Acronym for mandibular orthopedic repositioning appliance, a type of removable dental prosthesis with a modification to the occlusal surfaces used with the goal of repositioning the mandible to improve neuromuscular balance and jaw relationship.

16. Mucosal Insert

Any metal form attached to the tissue surface of a removable dental prosthesis that mechanically engages undercuts in a surgically prepared mucosal site also called button implant, intra-mucosal insert, mucosal implant.

17. Nesbit Prosthesis

Eponym for a unilateral partial removable dental prosthesis design, that De. Nesbit introduced in 1918.

18. Partial Denture

A removable dental prosthesis or a fixed dental prosthesis that restores one or more but not all of the natural teeth and/or associated parts and may be supported in part or whole by natural teeth, dental implant supported crowns, dental implant abutment(s), or other fixed dental prosthesis and/or the oral mucosa.

19. Partial Denture Retention

The ability of a removable dental prosthesis to resist movement away from its foundation area and/or abutments.

20. Path of Placement

The specific direction in which a prosthesis is placed on the abutment teeth or dental implant(s).

21. Removable Partial Denture Prosthesis

Any prosthesis that replaces some teeth in a partially dentate arch. It can be removed from the mouth and replaced at will, also called partial removable dental prosthesis.

22. Resilient Attachments

An attachment designed to give a tooth borne/soft tissue borne removable dental prosthesis sufficient mechanical flexion, to withstand the variations in seating of the prosthesis due to deformation of the mucosa and underlying tissues without placing excessive stress on the abutments.

23. Rest Seat

The prepared recess in a tooth or restoration created to receive the occlusal, incisal, cingulum or lingual rest.

24. Retentive Clasp

A clasp specifically designed to provide retention, by engaging an undercut. A flexible segment of a partial removal dental prosthesis that engages an undercut on an abutment and that is designed to retain the prosthesis.

25. Retentive Fulcrum Line

An imaginary line connecting the retentive points of clasp arms on retaining teeth adjacent to mucosa-borne denture bases. It is also known as clasp line; around which the removable dental prosthesis tends to rotate when subjected to dislodging forces.

26. Ring Less Investment Technique

An investing technique that uses a removable paper or plastic cylindrical outer form permitting unrestricted expansion of the investment by comparison to the use of a steel casting ring.

27. Rotational Path Removable Partial Denture

A partial removable dental prosthesis that incorporates a curved, arcuate, or variable path of placement allowing one or more of the rigid components of the framework to gain access to and engage an undercut area.

28. Semiprecision Attachment

A laboratory fabricated rigid metallic extension (Patrix) of a fixed or removable dental prosthesis that fits into a slot-type keyway (matrix) in a cast restoration, allowing some movement between the components.

29. Semiprecision Rest

A rigid metallic extension of a fixed or removable dental prosthesis that fits into an intracoronal preparation in a cast restoration.

30. Sprue

The channel or hole through which plastic or metal is poured or cast into a gate or reservoir and then into a mold.

31. Survey Line

A line produced on a cast by a surveyor marking the greatest prominence of contour in relation to planned path of placement of a restoration.

32. Surveying

An analysis and comparison of the prominence of intra-oral contours associated with the fabrication of a dental prosthesis.

33. Treatment Denture

A dental prosthesis used for the purpose of treating or conditioning the tissues that is called on to support and retain it. It is also known as interim prosthesis.

34. Undercut

The portion of the surface of an object that is below the height of contour in relationship to the path of placement.

35. Wax Addition Technique

The process used to develop a wax pattern through organized sequential addition of wax to shape the individual components of the desired anatomic form.

36. Wrought

Worked into shape by tools or formed.

37. Yield Strength

The strength at which a small amount of permanent (plastic) strain occurs, usually 0.1% or 0.2% and most frequently measured in MPa or Psi.

MULTIPLE CHOICE QUESTIONS

1. **Most common missing tooth in adult population is:**
   A. Mandibular first molar
   B. Maxillary first molar
   C. Mandibular second molar
   D. Maxillary second molar.

2. **Which of the following factor is most important for success with removable partial denture?**
   A. Retention
   B. Support
   C. Stability
   D. None of the above

3. **The Kennedy's classification system of partially edentulous arches fulfills following criteria *except*:**
   A. Permits immediate visualization of arches
   B. Differentiate between tooth and tooth-tissue supported prosthesis
   C. Allows logical approach to partial denture design
   D. Quantify amount of support from tooth and tissue.

4. **A Patient with high caries susceptibility and poor oral hygiene requiring replacement of missing teeth is best treated with:**
   A. Oral Implants
   B. Fixed partial dentures
   C. Removable partial dentures
   D. Complete dentures

5. **Cross arch stabilization, by bilateral removable prosthesis would be indicated over fixed prosthesis when:**
   A. Inter abutment span is large
   B. Pier abutment is present
   C. Excessive ridge undercuts present
   D. Reduced periodontal surface area

6. **The concept of shortened dental arch consist of:**
   A. Not replacing any missing posterior teeth
   B. Replacing few posterior teeth only
   C. Improves masticatory efficiency
   D. Prevents extrusion and migration of opposing tooth.

7. **Shortened mandibular arch when needing replacement for missing molar is best treated by:**
   A. Dental implant
   B. Removable partial denture
   C. Fixed cantilever prosthesis
   D. Left untreated

8. **Shortened maxillary arch when needing replacement for missing molar is best treated by:**
   A. Dental implant
   B. Removable partial denture
   C. Fixed partial denture
   D. Precision denture

9. **A 35-year old female patient with missing maxillary front teeth (Incisors) due to trauma 5 years back desires to replace her front teeth. The patient can be best treated with:**
   A. Conventional fixed partial denture with canine as abutments
   B. Cast removable partial denture
   C. Resin bonded prosthesis
   D. Oral implants with bone augmentative procedures.

10. **A patient wanting replacement of missing mandibular posteriors unilaterally but with third molar fully erupted and present in occlusion. The choice of prosthesis would be:**
    A. Fixed partial denture made in Co-Cr alloy
    B. Implant supported bridge
    C. Stress breaker prosthesis
    D. Cast removable partial denture.

11. **The prognosis of which of the following maxillary prosthesis against Class II (Retrognathic) mandible is best**
    A. Complete removable denture
    B. Cast removable partial denture
    C. Implant supported dentures
    D. None of the above

12. **Displaceability of mucoperiosteum (mucosa) and periodontal ligament is approximately respectively:**
    A. (1.0 mm), (0.25 ± 0.1 mm)
    B. (2.0 mm), (1 ± 0.1 mm)
    C. (3.0 mm), (6.5 ± 0.1 mm)
    D. (2.0 mm), (0.25 ± 0.1 mm)

NOTES

13. **A patient having both anterior and posterior separate edentulous space should ideally be replaced by:**
    A. Removable prosthesis both anteriorly and posteriorly.
    B. Fixed prosthesis both anteriorly and posteriorly.
    C. One prosthesis replacing anterior and posterior teeth.
    D. Anteriorly fixed prosthesis always.

14. **Which of the following is not a part of cast partial denture?**
    A. Rest seat
    B. Finish lines
    C. Retentive meshwork
    D. Proximal plate
    E. Guide planes

15. **For a mandibular RPD which of the following factors are arranged in correct order of importance:**
    A. Support > stability > retention > esthetics
    B. Retention > stability > esthetics > support
    C. Stability > retention > support > esthetics
    D. Stability > support > retention > esthetics

16. **The main disadvantage of extracoronal clasp retained partial denture over internal attachment denture is:**
    A. Esthetics
    B. Abutment stress
    C. Caries
    D. Bone loss

17. **Which of the following removable partial denture will need frequent reline?**
    A. Mandibular Kennedy Class II mod I
    B. Mandibular Kennedy Class I
    C. Maxillary Kennedy Class I
    D. Maxillary Class IV

18. **Which of the following factors do not form the basis of any classification system for partially edentulous situations?**
    A. Position and number of direct retainers
    B. Relationship of abutment tooth and alveolar ridge
    C. Periodontal condition of abutment teeth
    D. Location and extent of edentulous space
    E. Density of residual alveolar ridge bone.

NOTES

19. **Modification spaces in Kennedy's classification refers to:**
    A. Posterior most edentulous area
    B. Edentulous space bounded by periodontally weakened abutment
    C. Any space not to be included in designing
    D. None of the above

20. **A 54-year old male having missing 18, 17, 16, 15 and 24, 25 with 38, 48 impacted would be classified according to Kennedy classification as:**
    A. Class II   B. Class I
    C. Class III mod I   D. Class II mod I

21. **Tooth bounded edentulous situations are considered to be tooth supported whilst classifying for removable partial dentures for:**
    A. Up to maximum two missing teeth
    B. Up to four missing teeth
    C. Maximum 3 teeth missing
    D. Only one tooth missing

22. **The first system for classifying partially edentulous arches was given by**
    A. Kennedy   B. Bailyn
    C. Cummer   D. Applegate

23. **Any commonly used classification system for partially edentulous arches can not be a deciding factor in partial denture designing due to which of the following factor:**
    A. Need for retention varies
    B. Patients unrealistic esthetic requirements
    C. Classification system gives no idea of support
    D. All of the above

24. **Kennedy's Class IV have no modifications:**
    True/False

25. **Partially edentulous arches should be best classified after all mouth preparations are done:**
    True/False

26. **According to Kennedy Applegate classification, class V is an edentulous situation in which teeth bounding the edentulous space anteriorly and posteriorly are capable of total support of the prosthesis**
    True/false

NOTES

ANSWERS

NOTES

1 B Partially edentulous conditions are more common in maxillary arch. Maxillary first molars are most commonly missing.

2 C Lack of stability is the most common factor for failure of RPD. In maxillae lack of stability is 7 times more prevalent than lack of retention. In mandible lack of stability is 1.8 times more prevalent than lack of retention.

3 D

4 D Carious and periodontally weakened abutment are not reliable for support.

5 C,D Whenever there is periodontally weakened abutment present or long edentulous span present, missing teeth are best restored with either oral implants or partial removable prosthesis.

6 B,D Shortened dental arch consist of not replacing missing posteriors until required for maintaining contact with the opposing teeth.

It is based upon findings that by not replacing first or second or both molars unilaterally or bilaterally unless otherwise opposing molars are present, masticatory function is not jeoparadized to a greater extent.

7 A

8 B In maxilla, whenever possible tuberosity should be covered. If left uncovered tuberosity enlargement makes further occlusal treatment difficult. However, from the patients point of view dental implant can satisfactorily replace missing molar.

9 D

10 D Because of the long span, lateral and oblique forces on any prosthesis would be damaging to the natural teeth and residual ridge both, hence, cast partial denture would be a viable option if the patient consents because of cross-arch stabilization. Main factor is control of stresses generated by and on the prosthesis.

11 B The mandibular teeth exert an upward forward thrust on the maxilla in the mouth with retrognathic occlusion. Cast removable partial denture are better able to resist disbalancing forces.

12 D

13 D Esthetics is the primary reason for anterior tooth replacement. Esthetics is better obtainable with fixed prosthesis.

14 A,E Rest seat and guide planes are prepared surfaces on the abutment teeth which are contacted by rest and proximal plate respectively.

15 D

16 A

17 B

18 E

19 D

20 D

21 C   When more than 3 teeth are missing, it is considered to be both tooth and tissue supported prosthesis.

22 C

23 D

24 True

25 True

26 False

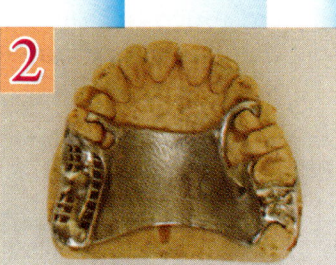

Component Parts of Removable Partial Denture

- ❏ Major connector
- ❏ Minor connector
- ❏ Rest
- ❏ Direct retainer
- ❏ Indirect retainer
- ❏ Denture teeth and denture base considerations
- ❏ Precision attachments and stress breaker

MAJOR CONNECTOR

A major connector is simply a component of removable partial denture which unites the components on one side of the arch to the components on the opposite side of the arch.

> Major connector is that structural unit of the partial denture to which all other parts are directly or indirectly attached.

Classification of Major Connector

Major connector can be simply classified as follows:
- I a. Maxillary major connector
  - b. Mandibular major connector
- II According to material
  - i. Metallic major connector
  - ii. Acrylic major connector (all acrylic palatal coverage).

Functions of Major Connector

- i. Major connector unifies and makes all other components effective.
- ii. It provides support and bracing of denture

iii. It aids in indirect retention
iv. It allows broad stress distribution between the teeth and mucosa.
v. Maxillary major connector also contributes to retention of the prosthesis.

General Requirements and Characteristics of Major Connector

i. Major connector should be rigid and provide cross-arch stabilization
ii. It should provide support and broad stress distribution.
iii. Major connector should be free of movable tissue and impingement of gingival tissue should be avoided (Figs 2.1A and B).

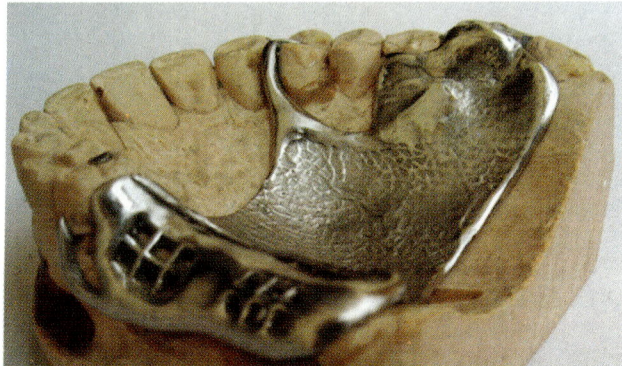

Fig. 2.1A: Borders of maxillary major connector should be 6 mm away from the free gingival margin

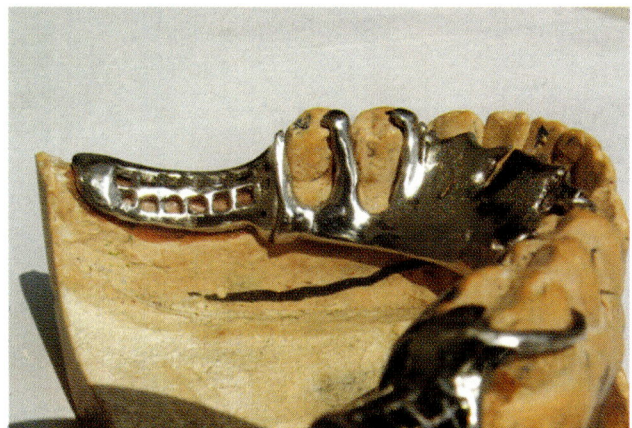

Fig. 2.1B: Borders of mandibular major connector should be minimum 4 mm away from the gingiva

Figs 2.1A and B: Borders of major connector should not impinge upon the gingival margins

Borders of mandibular major connector should be a minimum of 4 mm away from the gingival margin and that of maxillary major connector should be located 6 mm away from the gingival margin.

iv. Maxillary major connectors need no relief except in the area of palatal tori or median palatine suture.
v. Relief is generally required for soft tissue under mandibular major connector and where the framework crosses the marginal gingiva.
vi. Maxillary major connectors should be lightly beaded on the refractory cast (beading lines are created on master cast before duplication) to ensure intimate contact between the metal and palatal mucosa (Fig. 2.2).

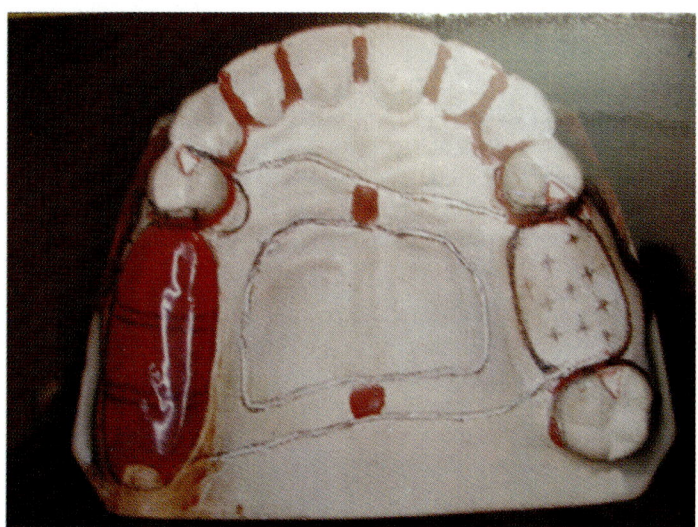

Fig. 2.2: Beading of Maxillary cast along the outline of major connector should be done as a shallow rounded V form groove 0.5 mm deep

vii. Major connector should not interfere with tongue or trap food particles.
viii. Major connectors should be made from alloy compatible with oral tissue.

Maxillary Major Connectors (Figs 2.3A to D)
Five basic type of maxillary major connectors are discussed (Table 2.1).

Mandibular Major Connectors (Figs 2.4A to C)
See Table 2.2 after Figs 2.3A to D.

Factor in Selection of Major Connectors (Table 2.3)
See Table after Figure 2.4A to C

Performance Ability of Major Connectors (Table 2.4)
See Table after Table 2.3.

	Type of Major connector	Structural details	Indications	Waxing specifications
		Table 2.1: Five basic type of maxillary major connectors		
1	**Single palatal bar**	• Less than 8 mm in width • Narrow half oval • Bulky • Uncomfortable to tongue	• No major indication besides replacing one or two teeth on either side of the arch • Interim partial denture	Half oval 6 gauge wax thickness.
2	**Single palatal strap**	• Minimum 8 mm or more • Sufficient rigidity without bulk • Cannot replace anterior teeth along with posterior missing teeth • Confined within an area bounded by four principal rests	• Bilateral short span tooth-supported edentulous area • Tooth supported unilateral edentulous area with cross-arch attachment through direct retainers	• Anatomic Replica pattern 22–24 gauge wax pattern
3	**Anterior-posterior strap**	• Parallelogram shaped • Anterior strap 8 to 10 mm located just posterior to rugae crest or in the valley between two crest. • Posterior strap is thin 8 mm wide located on the hard palate • Lateral or connecting straps are 7 to 9 mm wide and parallel to curve of arch.	• Suitable for almost all partial denture situations in maxilla • Class I and Class II arches with good abutment and ridge support • Class IV arches • Inoperable tori	• Anatomic Replica pattern form of 22 gauge wax thickness

4	**Complete palatal plate coverage**	• Excellent support rigidity and retention
		• Cannot be given when inoperable tori exists
		• Excessive tissue coverage can cause papillary hyperplasia and phonetic problems
		• Three design/variations are possible:
		  i. Complete cast metal plate extending up to the junction of hard and soft palate.
		  ii. Combination of cast metal plate anteriorly with resin extension posteriorly.
		  iii. All acrylic resin plate major connector.
			• When only some or all anterior teeth remains
			• Kennedy Class I and II situations
			• When both anterior and posterior teeth require replacement
			• Long edentulous span.
			• Poor ridge and abutment support.
				• Anatomic replica pattern of 22–24 gauge sheet wax thickness

5	**U-shaped palatal major connector**	• Lacks rigidity and support • Must be supported by occlusal rest and indirect retainers.	• Large inoperable tori extending posteriorly on soft palate. • Several missing anterior teeth.	• Anatomica replica pattern of 22–24 gauge thickness sheet wax.

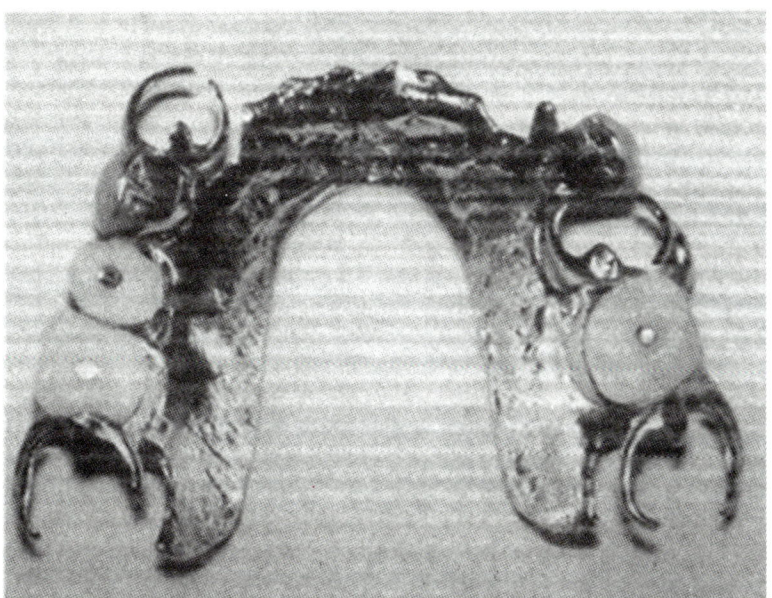

Fig. 2.3A: Horse shoe shaped

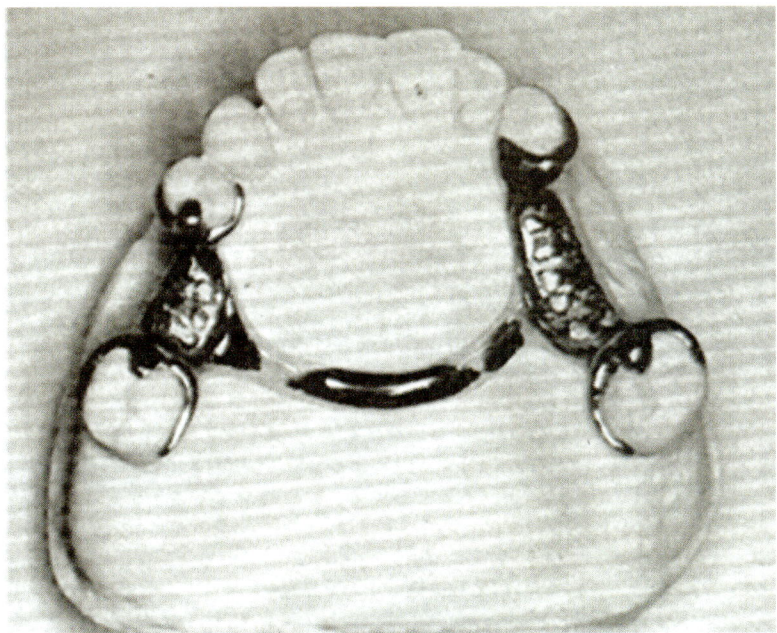

Fig. 2.3B: Palatal bar

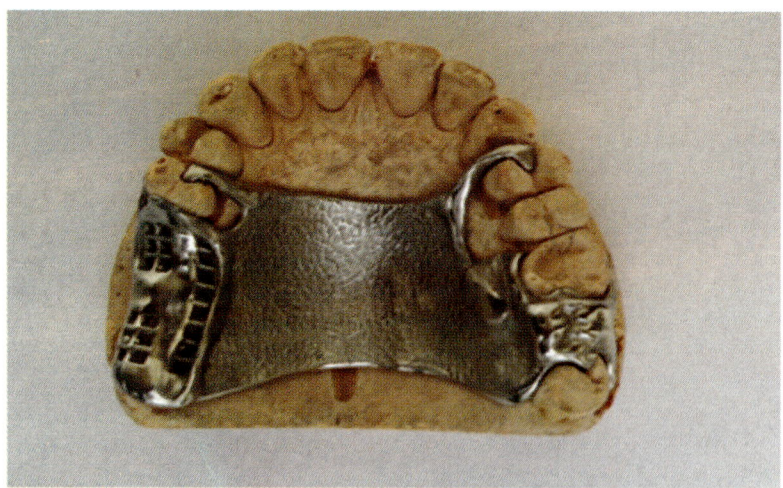

Fig. 2.3C: Single Broad palatal strap

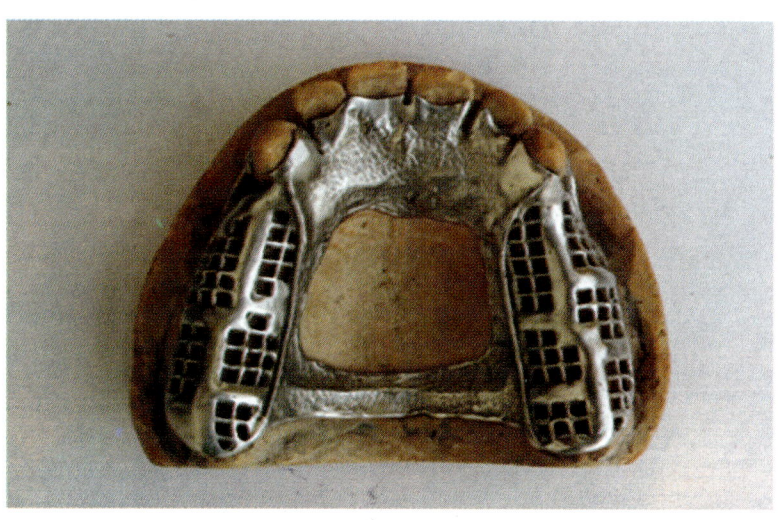

Fig. 2.3D: Anterior and posterior palatal strap

Figs 2.3A to D: Different types of maxillary major connector

Table 2.2: Mandibular Major Connectors (Figs 2.4A to C)			
Type of major connector	*Structural details*	*Indications*	*Wax specifications*
1 Lingual bar	• Superior border located minimum 4 mm away from free gingival margin • Inferior border half pear shaped located inferiorly at the functional floor of the mouth anteriorly in alveolar lingual sulcus	• Requires more than 8 mm of space between free gingival margin and functional floor of the mouth • All tooth supported situations • Cannot be used when lingual tori or lingual undercut exists.	• 6 gauge half pear-shaped wax pattern, can be reinforced with 24 gauge casting wax
2 Sublingual bar	• Requires specialised impression to record depth and width of lingual sulcus • The sublingual bar is more inferiorly and horizontally placed then lingual bar in the alveolar lingual sulcus. • The rigidity of sublingual bar is increased by a cube factor as the width increases.	• Sublingual bar can be used in lieu of lingual plate in the presence of anterior lingual undercut • It can be used in a shallow lingual sulci	• 6 gauge half pear shaped wax form reinforced with 22 to 24 gauge sheet wax
3 Linguo plate	• Inferior portion half pear shaped, bulkier, located inferiorly at the functional floor of the mouth. • It consist, of a thin metal collar extending superiorly from the inferior portion up to the supracingulum area. • In case of diastama, modification of linguoplate known as step back/cut back design is used. • Poor oral hygiene and decalcification may occur underneath	• Excessive posterior alveolar ridge resorption, as in Kennedys class I arches • Splinting of periodontally weakend teeth. • To provide indirect retention and horizontal stabilization of prosthesis. • When future replacement of one or more anteriors is anticipated.	• Inferior border 6 gauge half pear shaped wax form reinforced with 24 gauge sheet wax. • Superior apron 24 gauge sheet wax.
4 Continuous bar/double lingual/ Kennedy's bar	• Location same as lingual bar inferiorly • Superiorly, thin, narrow (3 mm) metal strap located on cingula of anterior teeth • Supported by rest on either side on principal abutment.	• Lingual inclination of anterior teeth demands blockout of interproximal spaces • When wide diastamata exists between mandibular anterior teeth	• Lingual bar 6 gauge half pear shaped wax pattern • Continuous bar pattern made up of two strips of 28 gauge sheet wax 3 mm wide.

Contd.

Type of major connector		Structural details	Indications	Wax specifications
5	Labial bar	• Superior border 4 mm away from labial and buccal gingival margin. • Inferior portion located in labial/buccal vestibule at the junction of attached and unattached mucosa. • Labial bar of hinged continuous connector (Swing Lock) is used as locking and retentive element.	• Excessive lingual tilt of anteriors and premolar teeth. • Severe lingual tori • Severe and abrupt lingual tissue undercut	• 6 gauge half pear shaped, reinforced with 24 gauge casting sheet wax.
6	Swing lock/hinged continuous bar	• It is a modification of linguo plate. • It consist of a labial bar that is connected to major connector by a hinge at one end and a latch on the other end. • It derives support from multiple rests on remaining natural teeth. • Stabilization is from linguoplate. • Retention is from bar type of clasp projecting from labial bar.	• Missing key abutments. • Unfavourable tooth contours. • Unfavourable soft tissue contours. • Teeth with questionable prognosis.	• Combination of labial bar and linguoplate wax pattern.

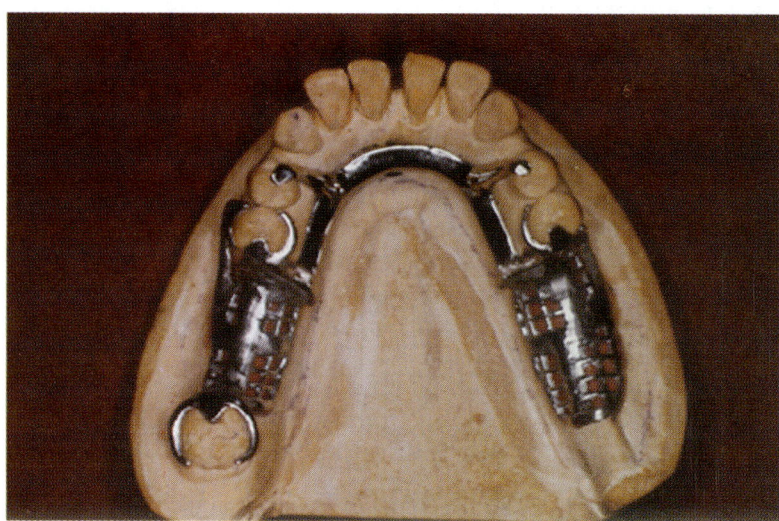

Fig. 2.4A: Linguo bar

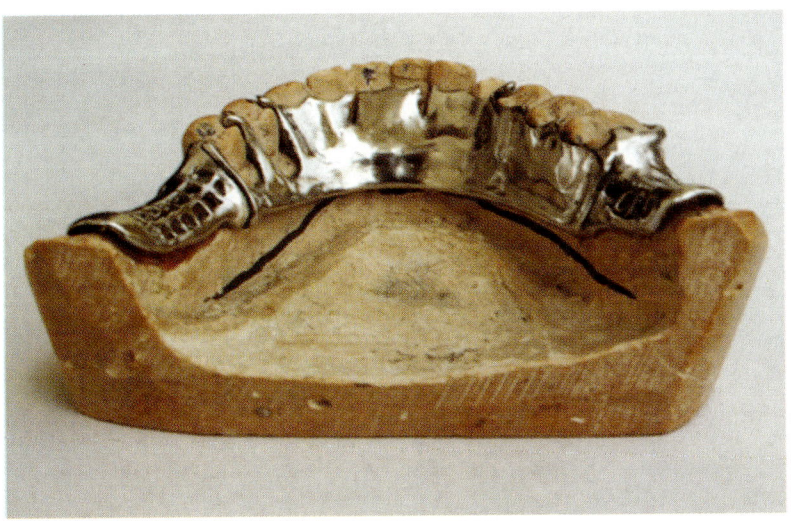

Fig. 2.4B: Lingual Plate

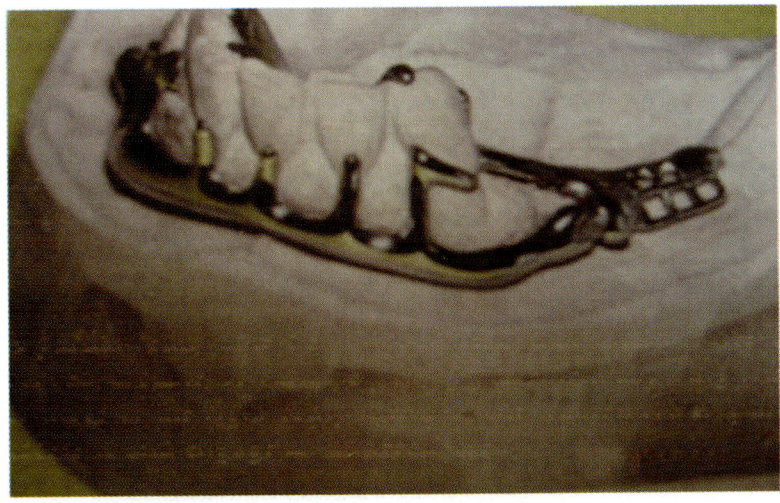

Fig. 2.4C: Labial bar

Figs 2.4A to C: Different types of mandibular major connectors

Table 2.3: Selection of major connectors		
Factor	Sailent feature	Choice of Major Connector
Selection of maxillary major connector is basically based upon the need for support		
1 Function (support, retention and stability)	• More the number of teeth missing or weaker periodontal support of remaining teeth, broader coverage of palate is required for maxillary major connector and vice versa	• Anterior and posterior strap when good abutment support exsist. • Complete palatal coverage when mucosal support is desired
2 Anatomical constraints	• Small tori can be covered with connector • Large lobulated torus should be circumvented	• Horse shoe connector and • Anterior-posterior bar can be considered when tori is present
3 Hygiene	• If coverage of the gingival margin is unavoidable, close contact between the connector and gingival margin should be achieved.	• Borders of the maxillary major connectors should be placed minimum of 6 mm away and parallel to the gingival margins so as not to compromise the blood supply.
4 Rigidity	• Palatal major connector when positioned in different planes can create an L beam effect.	• Anterior-posterior bar/strap creates a closed ring effect and ensures sufficient rigidity without compromising phonetics.
5 Patient acceptability	• It is best achieved by selecting a connector with minimal mucosal coverage without compromising the function.	Closed ring design major connectors are better tolerated than full coverage
Mandibular Major Connectors are selected primarily for the need of indirect retention		
1 Function (Need for Indirect attention)	• In mandibular arch mucosal support is less also rotation of denture along the fulcrum axis when dislodging forces are applied can lead to injury to mucosa anteriorly.	• Linguoplate and linguo bar major connector when supported by rest can control the downward anterior movement and provide indirect retention along with providing horizontal stability and stress distribution.
2 Anatomical consideration	• Inoperable tori • Lingual gingival recession • High lingual frenum attachment.	• Lingual bar should be at least 4 mm inferior to gingival margin. • If less than 8 mm exsist between gingival margin and functional floor of the mouth the choice of connector would be i. Linguo plate ii. a sublingual bar iii. a continuous bar • Labial bar may be considered when lingual tori exsist.
3 Patient acceptability	• No part of mucosa or teeth should be covered by framework unless indicated	• Lingual bars are better tolerated than linguo plate. Also, oral hygiene is better with lingual bar.

Table 2.4: Performance ability of major connectors		
Type of major connector	*Support*	*Rigidity*
Palatal strap	Good	Good
Complete palate	Excellent	Excellent
Anterior posterior	Poor	Good
Palatal bar	Poor	Poor
Horse shoe	Poor	Poor
Lingual bar	Poor	Good
Linguo plate	Poor	Good
Sublingual bar	Poor	Excellent

All Acrylic Denture (Figs 2.5A and B)

Acrylic dentures are most commonly indicated:

i. During the phase of **rapid bone resorption** following extraction

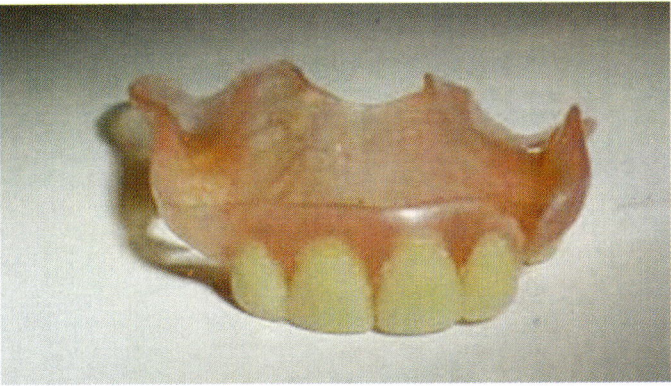

Fig. 2.5A

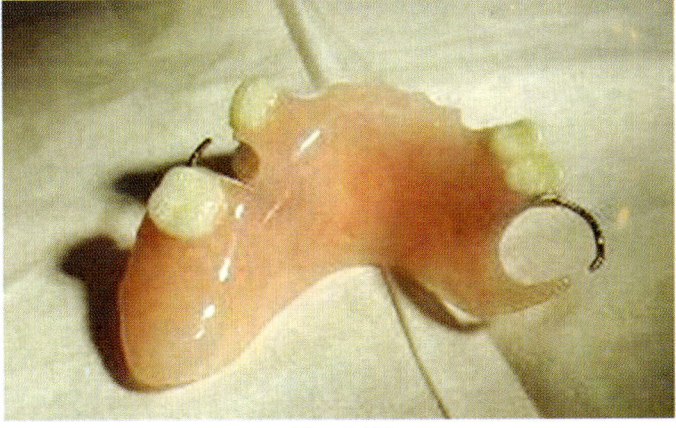

Fig. 2.5B

Figs 2.5A and B: All acrylic removable partial denture

ii. **Denture reline** as required in immediate denture

iii. **Transitional denture**: When the remaining teeth have a poor prognosis and their extraction and subsequent addition to the denture is anticipated.

iv. **Interim denture**: As a diagnostic denture (like assessing an increase in occlusal vertical dimension) before proceeding with fabrication of a definitive prosthesis.

v. **Young patients** where growth of the jaws and development of the dentition is not complete.

vi. When only a **few isolated** teeth remains, an acrylic connector may function just as effectively as one in metal.

Spoon Denture (Fig. 2.6)

i Is an all acrylic denture

ii Replaces one or two anterior teeth in young patient

iii. Reduced gingival margin coverage.

iv. Retention is by frictional contact between the acrylic connector and the palatal surface of some of the posterior teeth or by wrought wire clasp.

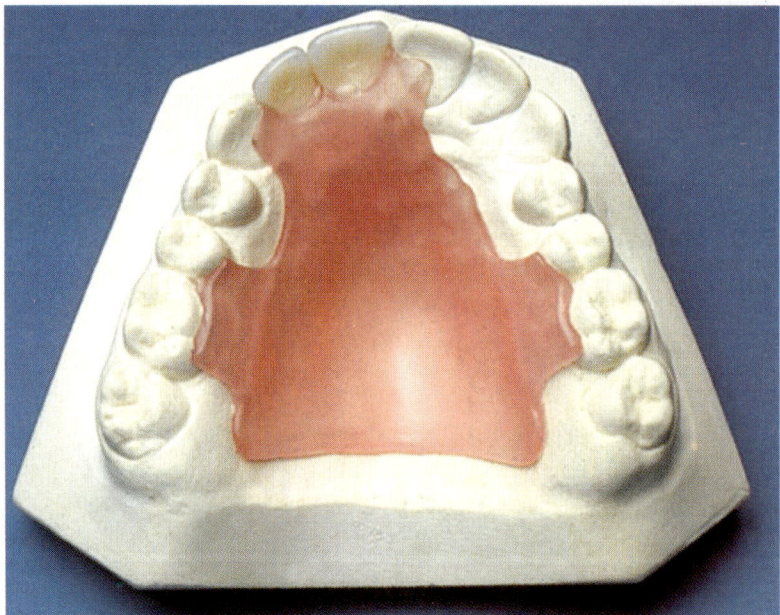

Fig. 2.6: Spoon denture

Every Denture (Fig. 2.7)

Is an all acrylic denture for restoring multiple bounded edentulous areas in the maxillary jaw. It has following characteristics.

i. Borders of connector at least 3 mm away from the gingival margins.

ii. Point contact between acrylic teeth and abutment teeth to reduce lateral stresses to minimum.

iii. Posterior wrought wire stops contributing to both denture retention and prevents distal drift of posterior teeth.

iv. Broader extension of flanges assist in bracing of the denture.

v. Balanced occlusion reduces lateral stress on the ridge.

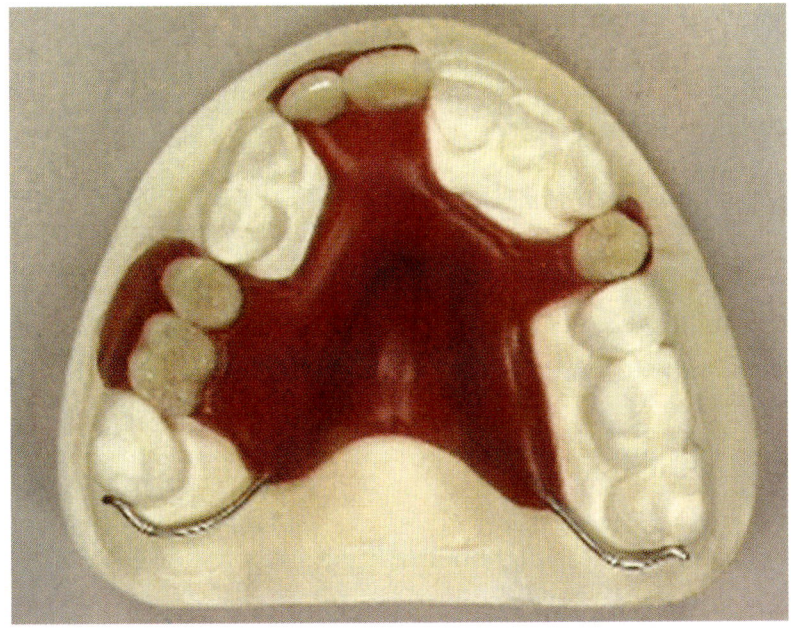

Fig. 2.7: Every denture

MULTIPLE CHOICE QUESTIONS

1. **Superior border of maxillary and mandibular major connectors should be located away from the free gingival margin minimum by:**
   A. 4 mm and 3 mm respectively
   B. 3 mm and 6 mm respectively
   C. 6 mm and 3 mm respectively
   D. 6 mm and 4 mm respectively

2. **Maxillary palatal strap when used as a major connector should be:**
   A. Minimum of 8 mm in width
   B. Borders should be beaded (0.5 mm)
   C. Replace few missing teeth on either side of the arch
   D. All of the above

3. **Linguoplate should be considered when the distance between the free gingival margin and functional floor of mouth is:**
   A. < 8 mm
   B. > 8 mm
   C. > 12 mm
   D. None of the above

4. **Major limitation in the usage of linguoplate as a major connector is:**
   A. Decreased support
   B. Inability to provide indirect retention
   C. Increased mobility of abutment teeth
   D. Risk of dental caries and plaque accumulation

5. **Maxillary major connectors are beaded at their borders so as to:**
   A. Prevent food debris accumulation beneath
   B. Intimate soft tissue contact
   C. Tapered round edges of connectors are comfortable to the patient
   D. Compensate for casting shrinkage
   E. All of the above

6. **The posterior border of complete palatal plate major connector should be:**
   A. Located at the junction of hard and soft palate
   B. Anterior to the junction of hard and soft palate

C. Posterior to the junction of hard and soft palate
D. Should incorporate posterior palatal seal

7. **Mandibular lingual bar half pear shape is made up of:**
    A. 4 gauge wax
    B. 6 gauge
    C. 24 gauge sheet wax
    D. Anatomica replica pattern

8. **Most rigid maxillary and mandibular major connector are respectively**
    A. Complete palate, sublingual bar
    B. Closed horse shoe, lingual bar
    C. A-P bar, labial bar
    D. Palatal bar, linguoplate

9. **Ring connector (anterior posterior palatal bar) have following limitations**
    A. Good rigidity
    B. Enhanced support
    C. L-beam effect
    D. Interference to tongue

10. **Sublingual bar is characterized by:**
    A. Located horizontally
    B. Located in the lingual sulcus at its maximum functional depth.
    C. Rigidity increases by a cube factor
    D. Can be used in place of linguoplate
    E. 6 gauge half pear shaped
    F. All of the above
    G. None of the above

11. **Flexible major connectors are indicated for:**
    A. Broad stress distribution.
    B. Indirect retention.
    C. Enhanced support
    D. Split major connector for stress breaking effect.

12. **Swing lock design partial denture have following characteristics**
    A. Labial bar as a retentive unit
    B. Linguoplate major connector.

C. Indicated when there are missing key abutments, and unfavorable soft tissue and tooth contours.

D. Contraindicated when lack of poor oral hygiene and plaque control exsist.

E. All of the above.

13. **Linguoplate should be used in preference to the lingual bar when**

A. Floor of the mouth and free marginal gingiva are > 8 mm apart.

B. Severe resorption of residual ridges and a distal extension RPD is required.

C. Periodontally strong anterior abutment teeth.

D. Indirect retention is not required.

14. **Apron of linguoplate should be:**

A. Scalloped contact with teeth

B. Placed below the survey line

C. Placed above the middle third of teeth

D. Thick and corrugated for rigidity.

15. **Sublingual bar is placed at floor of mouth. The following is not true about the sublingual bar.**

A. First suggested by Tryde and Brantenberg

B. 6 guage half oval

C. Placed in functional lingual sulcus

D. Greater in width then lingual bar.

16. **Selection of major connector are based upon all of the following factors *except*:**

A. Comfort

B. Rigidity

C. Location of denture base and support

D. Indirect retention.

E. Esthetics

17. **All acrylic removable partial denture are indicated as:**

A. Interim prosthesis

B. Treatment prosthesis

C. Transitional prosthesis

D. Definitive prosthesis

18. **Flexible acrylic partial denture is not an ideal method of replacing missing natural teeth because:**

A. Lacks cross arch stabilization

B. Lacks rigidity

C. Exerts lateral stresses leading to excessive residual ridge resorption

D. All of the above

19. Flexible all acrylic denture are best indicated:

A. Severe tooth and tissue undercuts in the path of placement

B. Replacement of tooth supported short span saddles

C. Microstomia

D. All of the above

E. Any partial edentulous situations

20. Relief under mandibular major connector is provided with:

A. 22 gauge wax B. 32 gauge wax

C. 26 gauge wax D. 6 gauge wax

21. Double lingual bar major connector is:

A. Indicated when interproximal spaces exists anteriorly

B. Space between free gingivae and floor of mouth is 8 mm

C. It consist of lower lingual bar

D. Upper bar is 2 to 3 mm in height

22. The double lingual bar major connector:

A. Also referred as "continuous lingual clasp"

B. Provides indirect retention

C. Provides horizontal stability

D. Wide distribution of stresses

E. All of the above

23. Salient features of Every denture are all *except*:

A. Restores multiple edentulous areas

B. Point contact between acrylic and abutment teeth

C. Broader extension of flanges

D. Balanced occlusion

24. The guide plane removal partial denture are used for:

A. Stabilizing teeth with poor bone support

B. Provide cross arch stabilization

C. Based upon broad stress distribution

D. All of the above.

25. Regarding swing lock removable partial denture following is correct:

A. Labial bar provides retention and stability.

B. Linguoplate provide support

NOTES

C. Ideally made up of gold alloys

D. Indicated for periodontally strong teeth.

26. **Which of the following is not the function of major connector?**
    A. Support
    B. Indirect retention
    C. Bracing
    D. None of the above.

ANSWERS

1 D

2 D

3 A

4 D

5 E

6 B   Because of the accuracy and stability of complete palate major connector conventional posterior palatal seal of maxillary complete denture is not required.

7 B

8 A

9 B

10 F

11 D

12 E

13 B

14 A

15 B

16 E

17 A   *Interim Prosthesis:* are those indicated for short period of usage till a more definitive prosthesis can be fabricated.

Treatment Prosthesis: Consist of a prosthesis which is used as a carrier for some medicament (Tissue conditioner) so as to enhance tissue recovery and healing without Jeopardizing the esthetic and function.

Transitional Prosthesis: Is a temporary restoration made to aid the patient in making a transition to complete denture when the total loss of teeth is inevitable.

18 D

19 All except E

20 B

21 All except B

22 E

23 A   Every denture restores multiple bounded areas only.

24 D   Broad stress distribution is the best method of obtaining support for weakened teeth. The stress is distributed through the use of rigid major and minor connectors, multiple rests and clasps.

25 A   First described by Dr. Joe J. Simmons in 1963. In Swing lock removable partial denture all or several of the remaining teeth are used to retain and stabilize the prosthesis.

Labial Bar is hinged and consists of vertical I bar projections on remaining natural anterior teeth. It provides retention and stabilization. Conventional linguo plate major connector provides path of insertion and removal.

26 D

MINOR CONNECTOR

Minor connector joins the major connector to the base of removable partial denture and other components such as the clasp assembly, indirect retainers, occlusal or cingulum rests.

Functions of Minor Connector

1. It joins various components of cast partial denture to the major connector.
2. It transfers functional stresses to the abutment teeth.
3. It transfers the effect of retainers, rests and stabilizing components throughout the prosthesis.

	Table 2.5: Location and types of minor connector	
	Location/Type	Function/Purpose
1	Embrasure between two teeth (Fig. 2.9)	• Joins the embrasure clasp or occlusal rest which is employed as indirect retainer to major connector • Should be triangular in form • Junction between the minor connector and major connector should be rounded • Should be wide buco-lingually but thin mesiodistally.
2	Proximal surface of abutment teeth/ guiding plane (Fig. 2.10)	• Gingivally proximal plate must extend from the marginal ridge to two thirds the length of crown. • Occlusally the outline form of proximal plate is triangular with apex located buccally and the base lingually. • Proximal plate minor connector provides reciprocation, stabilization and retention • The proximal plate should extend one half of the distance between tips of adjacent buccal and lingual cusp of the abutment teeth
3	Approach arm of bar/ Roach clasp (Fig. 2.11)	• It originates from the denture base area and places the bar clasp arm in the retentive undercut from the gingival direction • The terminal third of the approach arm should be flexible.
4	Minor connector providing attachment to resin denture base (Fig. 2.12)	• Minor connector for mandibular distal extension base should extend posteriorly upto $2/3$rd of the edentulous ridge • Minor connector for maxillary distal extension base should extend the entire length of the residual ridge up to the hamular notch. • Open lattice work or meshwork design is used. • Open lattice work provide enhanced retention for acrylic resin. Preformed 12 gauge half round and 18 gauge round wax is used for open lattice work.

Design Considerations for Minor Connector (Fig. 2.8)

1. Minor connector should be rigid and strong to withstand masticatory stresses and patient handling.
2. Minor connector should be positioned in the interproximal space, to avoid tongue interferences and should be thickest lingually and taper towards contacts area.
3. There should be a minimum of 5 mm of space between two vertical minor connectors.
4. Minor connector must contact the guiding planes surfaces of the teeth to facilitate a predictable path of placement for the removable partial denture.
5. Minor connector should cross gingival tissue abruptly and join major connector forming rounded right angle.

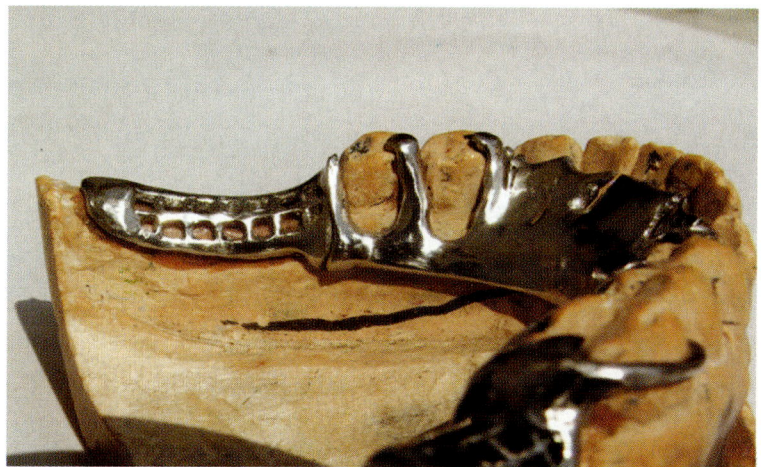

Fig. 2.8: Design considerations for minor connector: Minor Connector positioned in the interproximal space should taper towards the tooth . A minimum of 5mm should exist between two minor connector

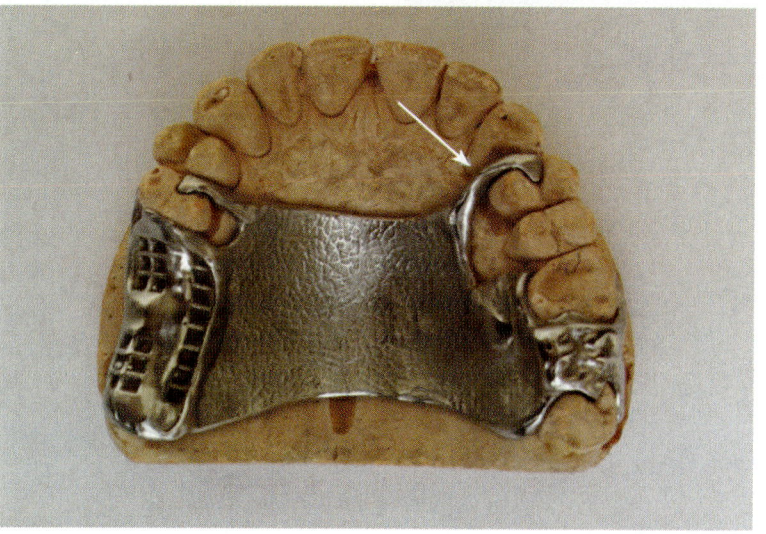

Fig. 2.9: Interproximal minor connector joins secondary occlusal rest to major connector (arrow)

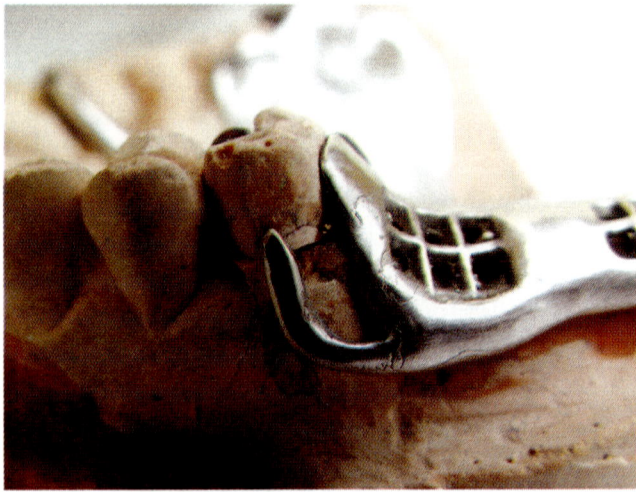

Fig. 2.10: Minor connector contacting the prepared guide plane

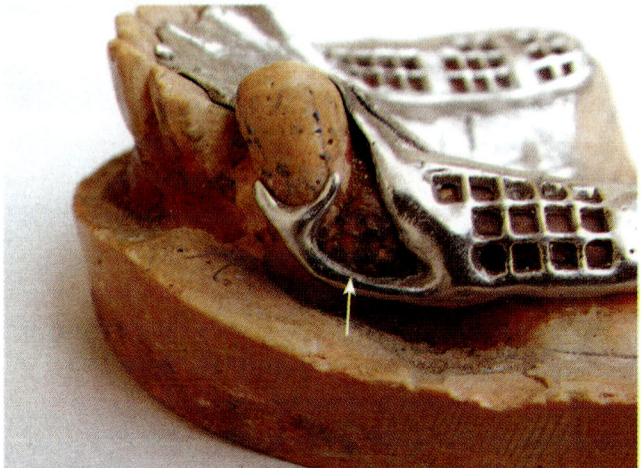

Fig. 2.11: Minor connector acting as approach arm of bar clasp

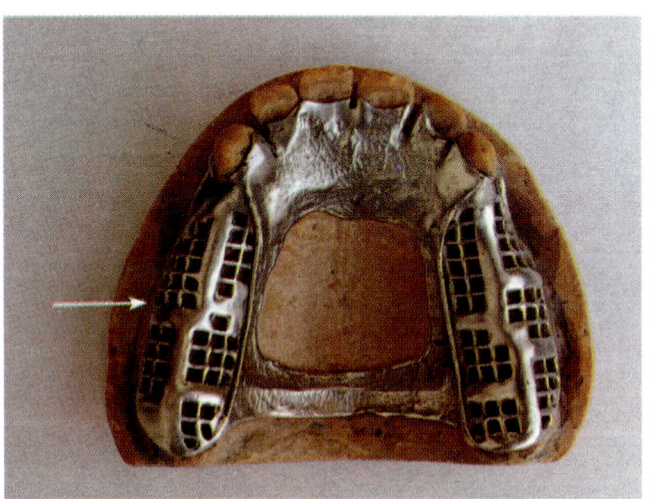

Fig. 2.12: Minor connector running over the saddle area and providing attachment to acrylic resin

Tissue Stops (Fig. 2.13)

   i. Tissue stops/tissue foot contact the residual ridge on the cast.
   ii. Provides stability to framework during transfer and processing.
   iii. Prevents framework distortion during packing of acrylic resin.
   iv. It is created in the metal framework by forming a small opening 2 × 2 mm in the saddle relief wax on the crest of the ridge prior to the duplication of the master cast.
   v. Finishing index tissue stop is designed to facilitate finishing of the denture base resin at the region of the terminal abutment by allowing positive contact of the metal framework with the cast ridge.

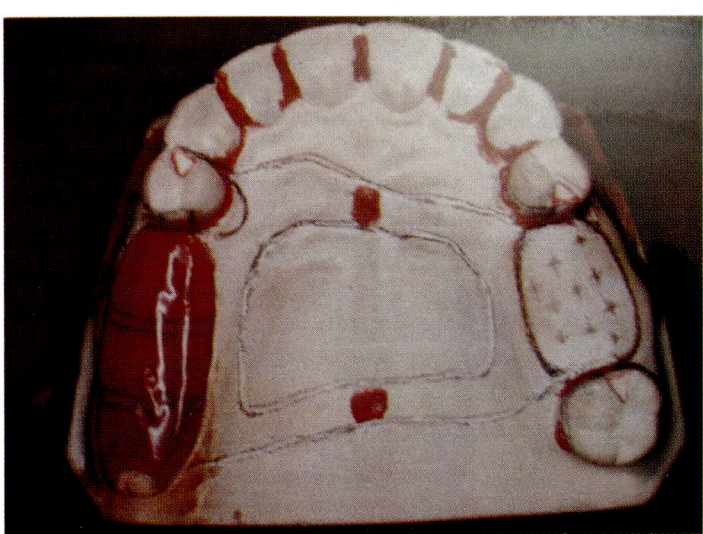

Fig. 2.13: Tissue stops formed by cutting out (2 by 2 mm) wax from relief wax at the distal end of the residual ridge on the master cast before duplication

Finish Lines (Figs 2.14A and B)

Finish lines are sharp, definite lines in the framework where the acrylic joins the metal, both on the tissue surface (internal finishing lines) and as well as on the polished surface (external finishing line) at the junction of denture base and the major connector.

External Finish Line (Fig. 2.14A)

Is formed at the wax up stage and should form an acute angle so that it creates a slight undercut in the metal. It

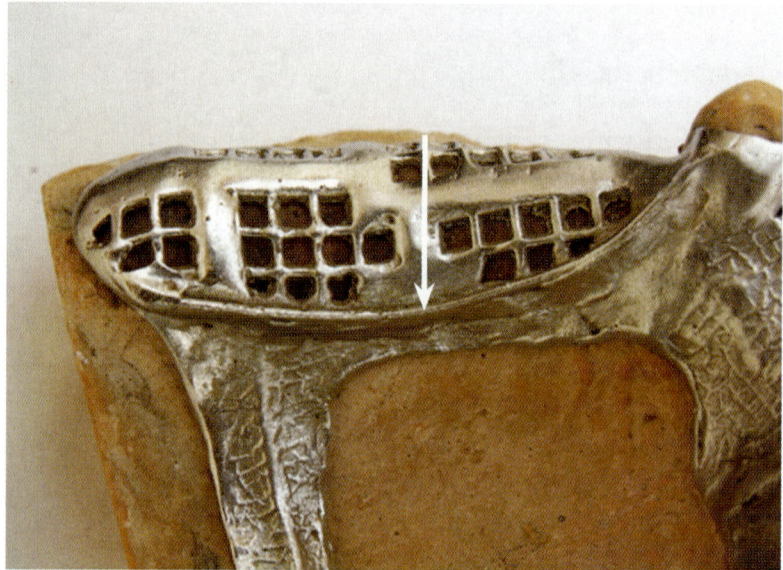

Fig. 2.14A: External finish line (arrow)

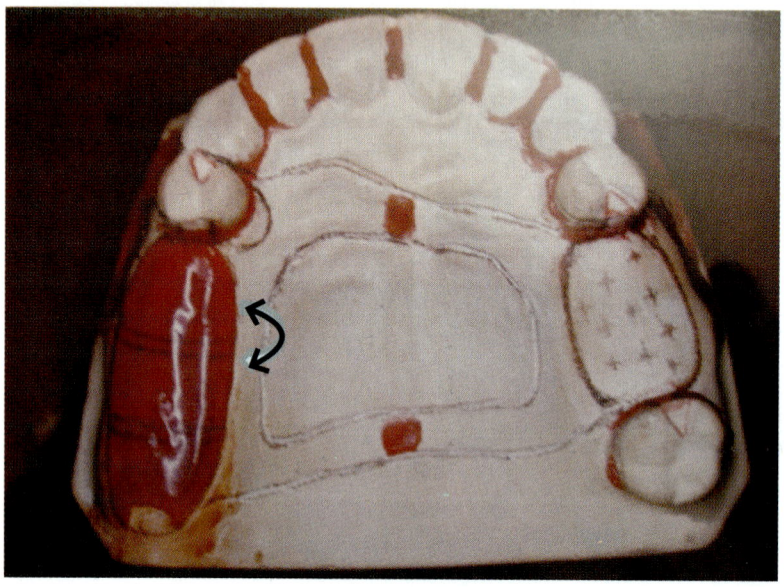

Fig. 2.14B: Internal finish line (arrow)

Figs 2.14A and B: Finish lines

should provide for sufficient thickness of metal and acrylic resin for strength and esthetics.

Internal Finish Line (Fig. 2.14B)

Is formed by the edges of saddle relief wax (24 gauge) placed on the master cast prior to the duplication.

MULTIPLE CHOICE QUESTION

1. **Metal bases are not recommended for distal extension situation because:**
   A. Need for frequent relining and adjustment
   B. Poor tissue tolerance
   C. Difficult to cast metal base
   D. Allergic tissue response

2. **For Kennedy Class III edentulous area with well formed ridge, choice of minor connector would be:**
   A. Open lattice work
   B. Mesh work
   C. Smooth metal base
   D. Metal base with retention aid for acrylic.

3. **Which of the following is not the function of finish lines?**
   A. Allows bulk of acrylic resin
   B. Create butt joint
   C. Reduce stress at the junction of metal and acrylic
   D. Prevents food trap beneath the saddle area.

4. **Finish line in the maxillary framework should be placed:**
   A. 2 mm palatal to the lingual contours of teeth.
   B. Over crest of the ridge
   C. Facial to the ridge
   D. None of the above

5. **Extension of mandibular minor connector over the edentulous ridge area in extension base partial denture should be:**
   A. One third the length of ridge
   B. Upto retromolar pad
   C. Three fourth the length of the ridge
   D. None of the above

6. **Proximal plate contact on the abutment tooth surface should be:**
   A. The entire proximal surface
   B. Up to the middle of middle third
   C. Upper one third only
   D. Junction of middle and the gingival third

7. **The junction of external finish line with the major connector should be:**
   A. > 90°   B. 90°
   C. < 90°   D. 180°

8. **Tissue stops are added in partial denture framework to:**
   A. Enhance support
   B. Provide retention
   C. Provide indirect retention
   D. Facilitate packing of resin

9. **Internal finish line results, from:**
   A. Wax-up on refractory cast
   B. Electrolytic polishing the finished denture
   C. It is carved by a carbide bur
   D. Relief wax placed on the master cast prior to duplication.

10. **Junction of major and minor connector should be:**
    A. U shaped   B. V shaped
    C. L shaped   D. Curved and smooth

11. **Minor connector joining claps assembly to major connector should be:**
    A. Positioned lingually in the middle of tooth
    B. Narrow buccolingually, broad mesiodistally
    C. Flexible
    D. None of the above

12. **Regarding lattice work minor connector which is not correct?**
    A. Provide strongest attachment to resin
    B. Facilitates relining and rebasing
    C. Can be used for replacing multiple missing teeth
    D. Consists of longitudonal strut placed over the crest of ridge

13. **Minor connector that contact the guide plane have following salient features** *except*:
    A. Half the distance between adjacent cusp tip
    B. Triangular in shape
    C. Extends gingivally from marginal ridge
    D. Part of clasp assembly

14. **Open lattice work is made up of:**
    A. 12 gauge half round wax
    B. 14 gauge round wax
    C. 16 gauge round wax
    D. 26 gauge half round wax

15. **Which of the following is not a function of minor connector?**
    A. Support   B. Bracing
    C. Stability   D. Predictable path of placement

ANSWER

1 A

2 D

3 D   Beading line or food line prevent food from undergoing beneath the partial denture.

4 A

5 D   Two third the length of ridge in mandible and entire length up to the hamular notch in maxillae.

6 D

7 C

8 D

9 D

10 D

11 D

12 D

13 D

14 A

15 A

REST AND REST SEAT

Rest are those components of a removable partial denture which transfers the forces along the long axis of abutment teeth, thereby providing support. Rest is a part of framework which fits into the prepared surface of abutment teeth known as rest seat. **Rests were first described by BonWill in 1899.**

Classification of Rests

1. **Primary rest** are basically part of retentive clasp assembly. They are the one's through which fulcrum axis passes. Their main function is to maintain predictable clasp position on the abutment.
2. **Auxillary/Secondary rest** serves to support the major connector or provide indirect retention. They are located opposite to fulcrum axis and away from the edentulous area.

> For the best mechanical advantage, the primary rest must be located closer to the edentulous area and the auxillary rest away from the edentulous area.

Purpose of Rest

Selection of rest area, the number of rests and depth of rest seat located in the abutment tooth is governed by patients oral musculature, amount of attrition, and according to biomechanics of the edentulous state.

Rest serves following purpose when properly utilized.

 i. The rest acts as a stop, prevents soft tissue injury under partial denture base and provides support.
 ii. Rest maintains the retentive terminal of the clasp in its intended position.
 iii. Auxillary rests serves as indirect retainer for distal extension partial denture.
 iv. Rest deflect food away from the area of contact between denture and tooth.
 v. It maintains occlusal contact and prevent extrusion of abutment teeth.
 vi. Rest can close a small space between teeth by bridging that space with back to back rest to restore arch continuity.
 vii. Rest provides rigid reciprocation to the retentive clasp arm.

A metal rest should never be placed on a tooth that is not prepared to receive it, otherwise inclined plane effect or slippage will occur.

Types of Rest (Table 2.6)

There are basically three main types of rest depending upon the location on tooth surface.

Table 2.6: Types of rest	
Type	*Salient features*
Occlusal rest (Figs 2.15A to C)	i. Occlusal rest should be placed in the greatest bulk of the tooth. The floor of the rest should be perpendicular to the long axis of the tooth ii. The outline form should be rounded triangular with the apex towards the centre. The floor of the rest should be spoon shaped. iii. Buccolingual width of the occlusal rest should be half the distance between cusp tips. Mesiodistally it should be one-fourth the length of the crown. Proximo-occlusal line angle should be rounded and the marginal ridge reduced by minimum 1.5 mm to ensure adequate bulk of metal. iv. Occlusal rest should be wide and thin not narrow and thick with the floor apical to the marginal ridge. There should be no sharp angles.
Cingulum rest (Fig. 2.16A and B)	i. Cingulum rest is closer to the centre of rotation of tooth and hence, exerts less leverage. A canine is much preferred over incisors for cingulum rest. ii. Lingual rest is inverted V shaped with the apex located incisally. The floor of the rest seat should be toward the cingulum and parallel to path of placement. iii. Mesiodistal length of preparation should be a minimum of 2.5 to 3 mm and should be crescent shaped. Labiolingually, width should be of 2 mm and incisal-apical height a minimum of 1.5 mm.
Incisal rest (Fig. 2.17)	i. Incisal rests are indicated on mandibular canines when cingulum rest is difficult to make. ii. Incisal rests may be placed on incisors for the purpose of stabilization and splinting. iii. An incisal rest seat should approach from the lingual surface cross the incisal edge and extend onto the facial surface of an abutment. iv. It is prepared like a V shaped notch located 1.5 to 2.0 mm from the proximal incisal angle of the tooth with the deepest part in the centre.
Other Types/form of Rest	
Rest on rotated tooth	Full coverage restoration should be planned with proper recess for rest. Full coverage restoration corrects the axial tooth contours and provides support for rest.
Quasicingulum rest	It is prepared for mandibular first bicuspids having rudimentary lingual cusp and consist of accentuated cingulum rest seat prepared in wax up of retainer which is bonded to the tooth after casting
Indirect retention rest (Fig. 2.18)	i. Also known as secondary or accessory rest, prepared commonly in the mesial fossae of the first bicuspid. ii. Located as far anterior and perpendicular to fulcrum line, as possible. iii. It consist of occlusal rest with canine extension.

Mesially inclined molar	The rest seat in mesially inclined molars should be prepared with the floor perpendicular to the long axis. Also, additional distal rest is placed occlusally for support.
Embrassure rest/ Interproximal occlusal rest (Fig. 2.19)	It is two occlusal rest joined interproximally. It prevents interproximal food wedging. It is usually indicated when there is no modification space present in Kennedy class II situation and the removable partial denture needs to be extended to the contralateral side for bilateral stabilization.
Onlay rest (Fig. 2.20)	i. Restores the occlusal plane of abutment tooth ii. Provides vertical support iii. The disadvantage is decalcification of tooth structure under the onlay rest seat.
Extended occlusal rest	i. Consists of extended occlusal rest extending more than one half the mesiodistal width of the tooth. It is approximately one-third the buccolingual tooth width. ii. It is indicated on mesially tipped most posterior molars next to modification space in Kennedy class II, or posterior abutment in Kennedy class III iii. It transmits forces along the long axis and ensures maximum bracing.

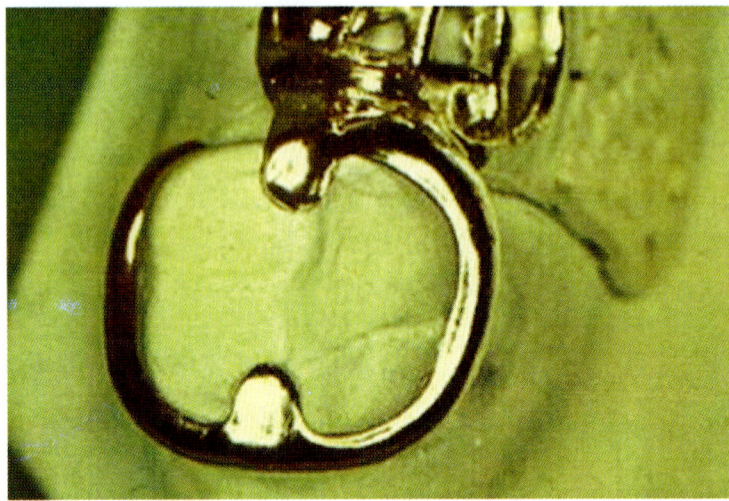

Fig. 2.15A

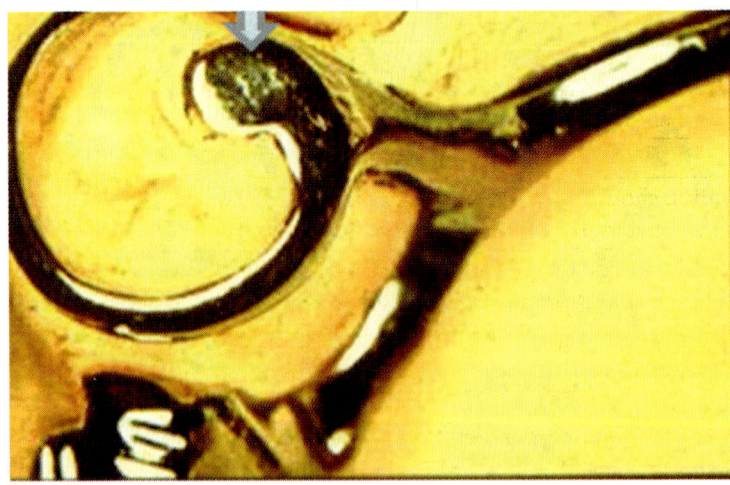

Fig. 2.15B

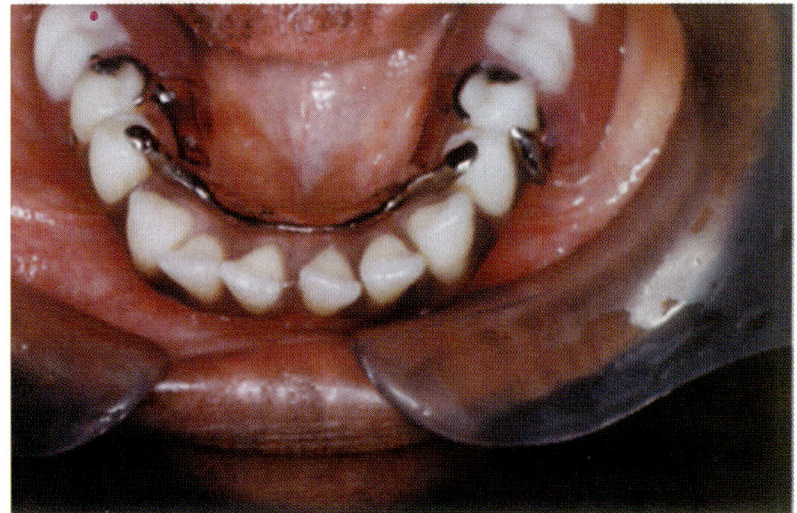

Fig. 2.15C

Figs 2.15A to C: Occlusal rest: Occlusal rest provides support and is placed in the greatest bulk of the tooth

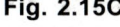

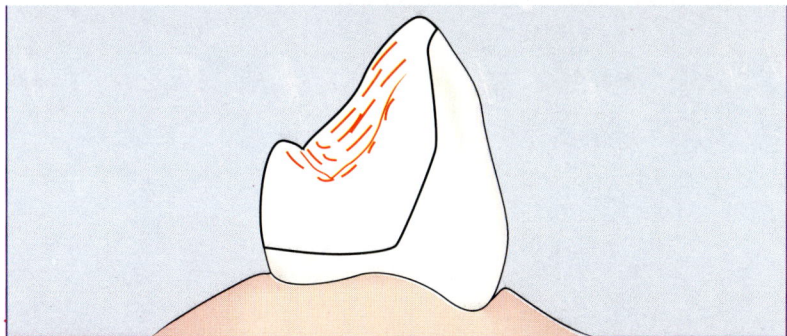

Fig. 2.16A

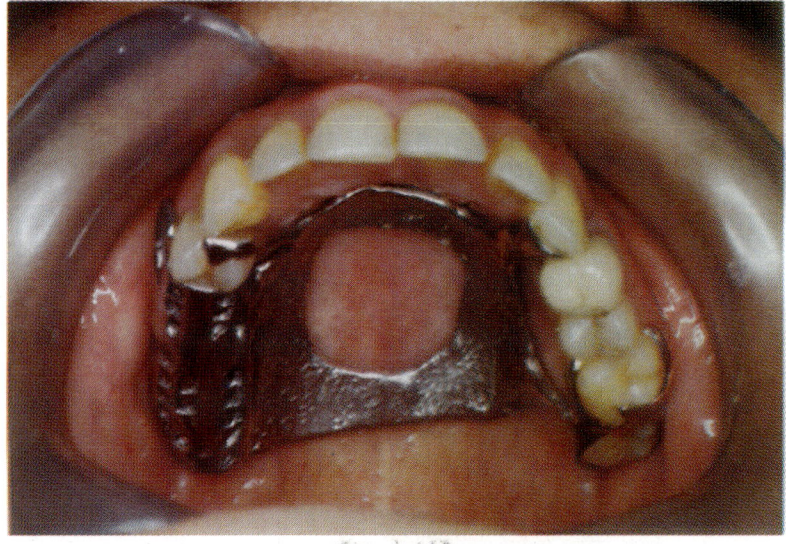

Fig. 2.16B

Figs 2.16A and B: Cingulum Rest: It is inverted V shaped with the apex located incisally, the floor of the rest is towards the cingulum and parallel to path of placement

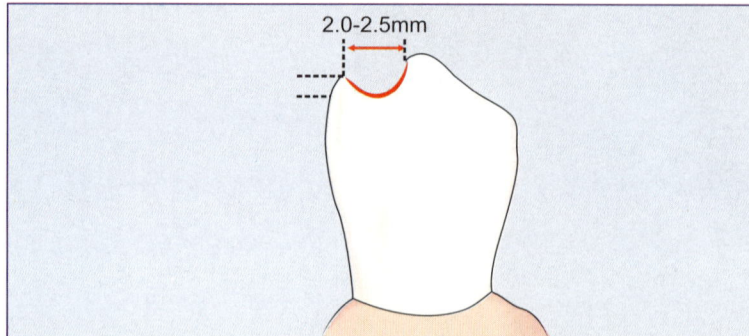

Fig. 2.17: Incisal rest: It is prepared like a V shaped notch located 1.5–2mm from the proximal incisal angle of the tooth with the deepest part in the centre

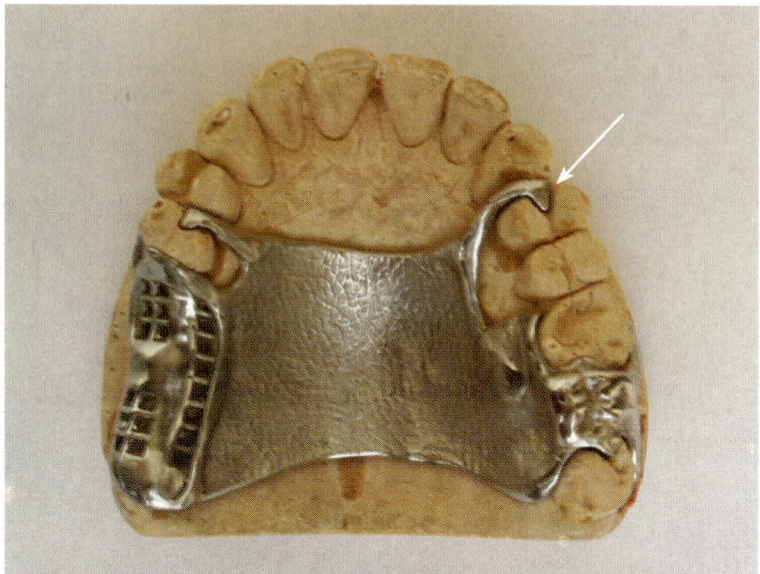

Fig. 2.18: Indirect retention rest (see arrow)

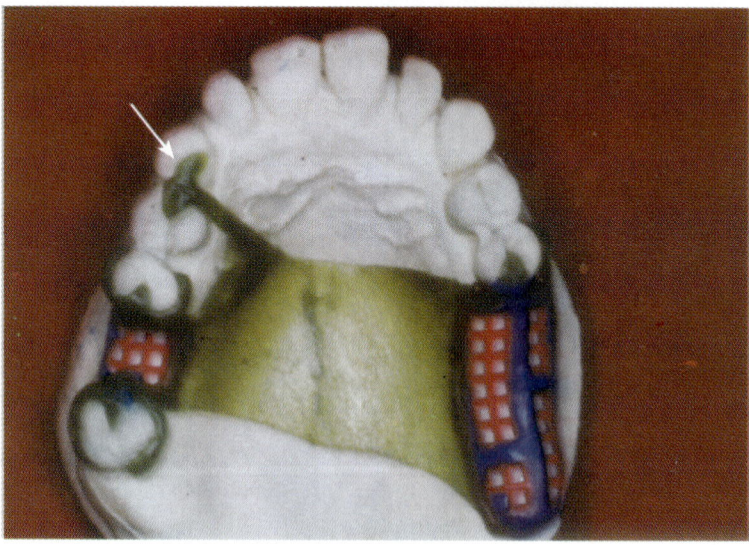

Fig. 2.19: Embrasure / Interproximal occlusal rest (see arrow)

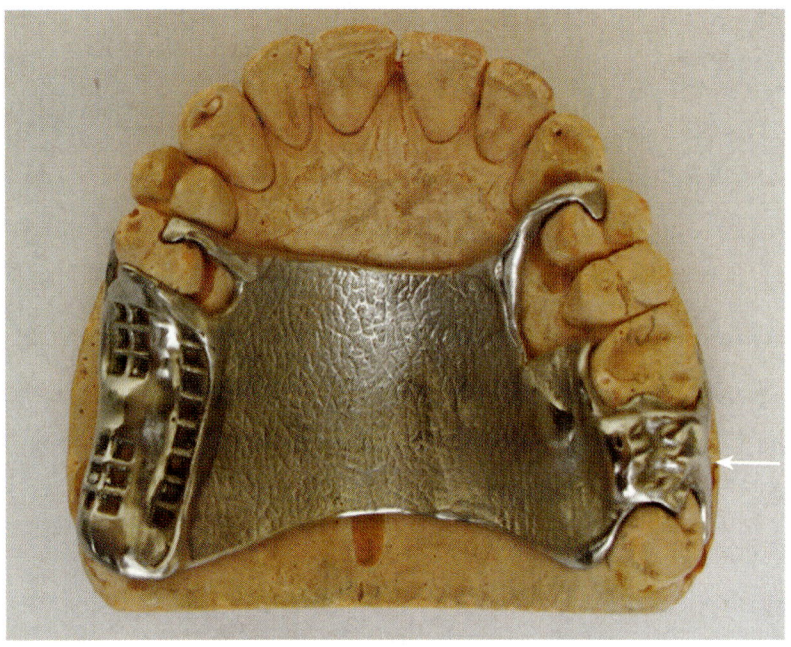

Fig. 2.20: Onlay rest (see arrow)

FOUNDATION/SUPPORT FOR REST

i. Rest should always be placed in a prepared recess in sound enamel or on any restorative surface that is capable of withstanding forces and resisting fracture and distortion thereby providing adequate support.

ii. Gold alloy is the most ideal surface to place rest seat followed by sound tooth enamel, fused porcelain, silver amalgam and composite resin.

iii. Whenever dentin is breached while preparing rest seat it should always be polished and covered with restorative material.

iv. Full coverage retainers may house occlusal or other rests when the abutment contours need improvement or modifications.

v. Occlusal rest seat in crowns and inlays are deeper than those made in natural tooth enamel.

vi. Occlusal rest on abutment in distal extension situations should be ball and socket to permit some movement of rest in rest seat. For tooth-supported dentures, the rest seat may be box like, also known as internal rest.

MULTIPLE CHOICE QUESTIONS

1. **The main function of occlusal rest in distal extension partial denture is:**
   A. Support
   B. Resist lateral forces
   C. Retention
   D. Cross-arch bracing

2. **The angle formed between the occlusal rest and the minor connector joining it to the framework is:**
   A. 90°
   B. <90°
   C. >90°
   D. 120°

3. **Onlay rests are indicated when/for:**
   A. Single tooth modification space
   B. Abutment in infraocclusion
   C. Abutment in supra occlusion
   D. None of the above

4. **Which of the following is not true for an occlusal rest?**
   A. Triangular outline with apex near center of the tooth
   B. Buccolingual width approx ½ the cusp distance
   C. The rest seat floor at the proximal end should be lower than the center.
   D. At least 1 mm thick.

5. **The preparation of rest seats should follow all selective grinding procedures:**

   True/False

6. **Which of the following is the function of extracoronal rest?**
   A. Orientation of metal framework to abutment teeth
   B. Predictable clasp positioning
   C. Indirect retention
   D. Prevents soft tissue trauma
   E. All of the above
   F. None of the above

7. **Rest seats are ideally created in:**
   A. Sound enamel
   B. Dentin
   C. Enamel dentin junction
   D. Restoration

8. **Ideal Restorative material for locating rest seat is:**
   A. Gold
   B. Amalgam
   C. Composite
   D. Glazed porcelain

9. **Trans occlusal rests are:**
   A. Occlusal rests that transverse occlusally between adjacent teeth
   B. Also known as back to back or double occlusal rests
   C. Prevents wedging action
   D. Provides additional support
   E. All of the above

10. **The floor of the occlusal rest seat should be:**
    A. Convex
    B. Located in dentin
    C. Perpendicular to the long axis
    D. All of the above

11. **Positive seat is:**
    A. Deepest portion of rest seat
    B. Concave
    C. 0.5–1 mm deeper
    D. All of the above

12. **The marginal ridge area is the most common site for rest fracture. It should be:**
    A. Reduced minimum by 1.5 mm
    B. Well rounded convex
    C. Reduced by 2.0 mm
    D. Prepared deeper than the apex

13. **The best method for checking the adequacy of prepared rest seat is:**
    A. Visual inspection
    B. Direct tactile contact
    C. Wax pattern
    D. Diagnostic cast

14. **Complete seating of the removable partial denture framework over abutment is determined primarily by:**
    A. Tooth contact of shoulder and terminal arm
    B. Complete seating of occlusal rest
    C. Proper adaptation of denture base to residual ridge
    D. Proper positioning of major connector

NOTES

15. **Incisal hook rest seat is given on mandibular canines. The main advantage is:**
    A. Esthetics
    B. Enhanced retention
    C. Greater stability
    D. All of the above

16. **Which of the following is not true with respect to cingulum rest?**
    A. Slopes cervically at line angles of cingulum
    B. Base of the rest is convex
    C. 1.5 mm deep
    D. Mostly given on maxillary canines

17. **Lingual ledge rests are indicated for:**
    A. Tilted molars
    B. Mandibular anteriors
    C. Maxillary anteriors
    D. Maxillary molars

18. **Lingual rest seats are:**
    A. Placed on crown restorations
    B. Located cervically to avoid interferences
    C. Placed perpendicular to the long axis.
    D. All of the above

19. **Occlusal rest preparation is done with:**
    A. Pear shaped bur
    B. Straight
    C. Oblong shaped bur
    D. Round bar

20. **Occlusal rest seats placed in crowns and inlays are generally larger and deeper than those in enamel:**

    True/False

21. **Occlusal rest made in abutment crowns for tooth-tissue supported dentures are deeper and box like internal rests:**

    True/False

NOTES

ANSWERS

1 A The relation of the occlusal rest to the abutment tooth should simulate a shallow ball and socket joint. Components of RPD other than the occlusal rest must be used to resist horizontal or oblique destructive forces.

2 B

3 B Onlay rests are most often used to restore the plane of occlusion and the occlusal morphologic features of the tooth. They can be used on multiple teeth for restoring plane of occlusion. Main disadvantage is high incidence of dental caries beneath onlay rest.

4 C The rest seat should be lower at the centre (apex) and higher at the marginal ridge (proximal end). When viewed laterally an occlusal rest should be spoon shaped. The occlusal surface of rest should be concave.

5 (True) If the rest seats are prepared first then procedures for creating guide planes or to lower survey lines would alter the character of the rest preparation.

6 E

7 A

8 A Gold and gold substitutes are the most acceptable restorative material to support rests.

9 E

10 C

11 D

12 A, B

13 D

14 B

15 C Incisal hook rest seats are prepared as a modifications of the incisal rest seat. It extends for an additional 1.5 to 2 mm as a concave depression on the labial surface. The main advantage of incisal hook is greater stability over incisal rest.

16 B

17 C The lingual ledge rest is usually employed on anterior teeth without a cingulum or on anterior teeth with a cingulum that is rudimentary.

18 D

19 D

20 (True)

21 (False) For tooth-tissue supported dentures occlusal rests are ball and socket joint type.

DIRECT RETAINER

Definition: A clasp/direct retainer is that component of the removable partial denture prosthesis that engages an abutment tooth to resist displacement of the prosthesis away from basal seat tissue.

Purpose of Direct Retainers/Clasp

i.   Clasp fits against the vertical enamel surface of an abutment tooth and provides frictional resistance to dislodging forces.
ii. Rigid reciprocal arm provides bracing and stability. Where as, flexible retentive arm tip engages undercut on abutment teeth to provide primary retention.
iii. Clasp helps in controlling lateral forces and distributes the forces between abutment teeth and adjacent edentulous ridge by accommodating functional movements in distal end situations.
iv. Stress breaking and equalization role of clasp helps in preservation of residual alveolar ridge and remaining teeth.

Types of Direct Retainers

Direct retainers are basically classified as:
I.   **Intracoronal:** Internal or precision attachment
II. **Extracoronal:** Clasp assembly or external attachment.

Intracoronal Direct Retainers

i.   First introduced by Herman E.S. Chayes in 1906.
ii.   Retention is by frictional means and by binding of components.
iii. It consist of either prefabricated precision or casted components in the form of male (part of denture) and female assembly which is contained within the contours of a fixed restoration on the abutment tooth.
iv.   It is more esthetical, as visible clasp arm is eliminated.
v.   Requires long clinical crown and cannot be done on young teeth due to high pulp chamber.
vi.   They are difficult to repair.
vii. They are costlier and requires precise laboratory procedures.

Extracoronal Direct Retainers (Figs 2.21A and B)

i. They are either clasp assemblies as described first by **Dr. W.G.A. Bonwill** in 1899 or as extracoronal attachments first introduced by **Henry R. Boos**.

ii. The clasp type retainer uses a flexible clasp arm engaging an undercut or depression on external surface of abutment tooth for retention.

iii. Extracoronal attachments uses interlocking components or spring loaded devices that engages a tooth contour to resist occlusal displacement.

iv. **Dr. Edward Kennedy** 1928 described the greatest circumference of a tooth as **Height of Contour**.
   M.M. Devan described the surface of tooth above the height of contour as suprabulge and that below as infrabulge.

v. Extracoronal direct retainers those approaching the undercut from suprabulge area are referred to as **Aker's/Circumferential clasp**.

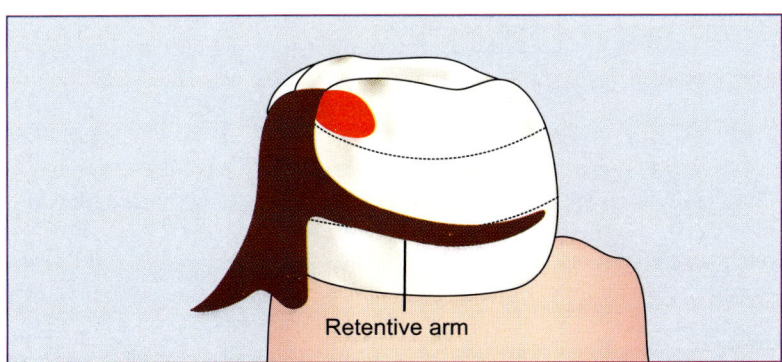

Fig. 2.21A: Suprabulge clasp

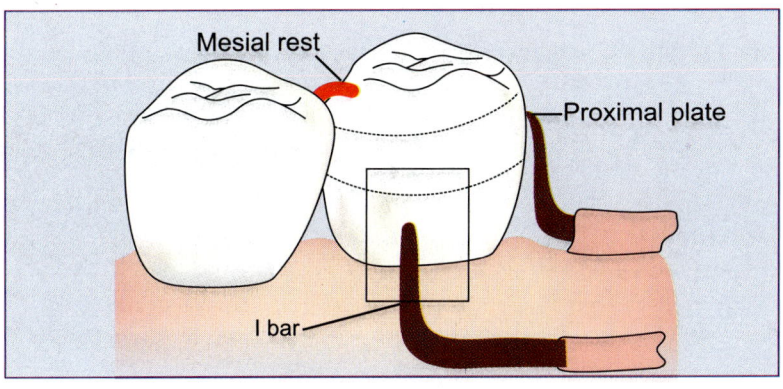

Fig. 2.21B: Infrabulge clasp

Figs 2.21A and B:
Extracoronal direct retainers

vi. Extracoronal direct retainers those approaching the undercut from infrabulge area are referred to as **Roach/Bar type clasp**.

Structure/Parts of a Clasp Assembly (Table 2.7) (Fig. 2.22)

A clasp assembly consists of following parts:
1. Rest
2. Retentive arm
3. Reciprocal arm
4. Minor connector/approach arm

Table 2.7: Parts of clasp assembly and their functions	
Parts of clasp assembly	*Function/Purpose*
Rest (occlusal/lingual/incisal)	i. Located on occlusal one third of tooth surface ii. Provides support and resists displacement of clasp in a gingival direction iii. Prevents the clasp arms from spreading iv. Maintains clasp in a predictable predetermined position

Retentive arm	i. Located in the gingival third in the desired undercut (below the height of contour)
	ii. They are either suprabulge as in circumferential clasp or infrabulge as in bar clasp
	iii. Suprabulge retentive arm arises from the minor connector and consist of; body → shoulder → retentive arm and retentive tip
	iv. Body and shoulder are rigid whereas the retentive arm gradually tapers down from its point of origin to retentive tip which is the only flexible part of the retentive arm and is located in the undercut
	v. Infrabulge retentive arm consists of:
	  a. **The approach arm:** Flexible minor connector originating from the framework, travels horizontally before crossing the free gingival margin at 90 degrees
	  b. **The retentive tip:** Arise from the vertical portion of minor connector and engages the predetermined undercut.

Reciprocal arm	i. It is located in the middle of middle third and on the surface of the tooth opposite to the retentive arm. ii. It provides horizontal stability and counter balances the stresses generated by the retentive arm. iii. Reciprocal arm should contact the abutment slightly before the retentive arm during insertion and should contact the opposing tooth surface till the retentive arm is completely seated. iv. Abutment surface to be contacted by the reciprocal arm should be prepared parallel to path of insertion and removal.
Minor connector (synonym: trussarm, tail, tang, upright)	i. It unites the body and clasp arms to the remainder of the framework and acts as a guiding plate to direct insertion and removal of the prosthesis. ii. It can act as a reciprocal element to counteract the forces generated by the retentive arm. iii. It can also act as an approach arm for infrabulge clasp.

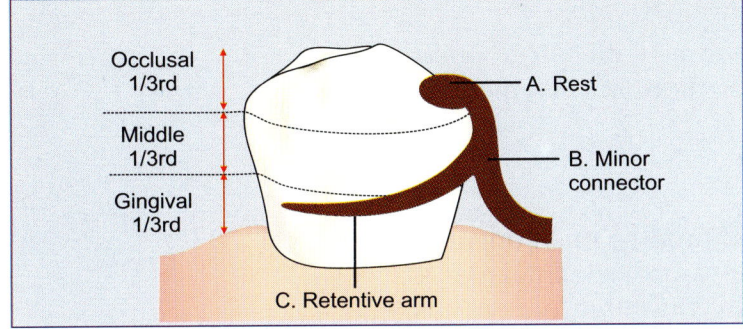

Fig. 2.22A

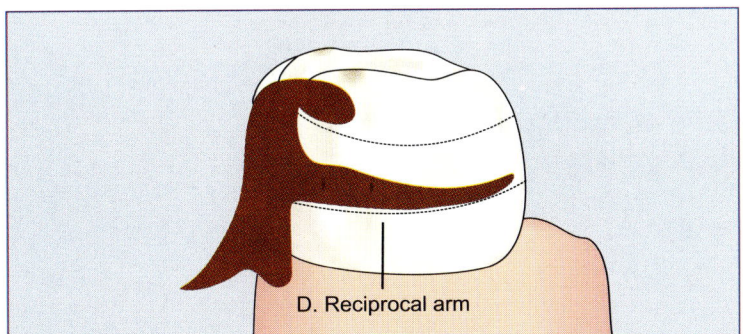

Fig. 2.22B

Figs 2.22A and B: Parts of clasp assembly (A) Rest (B) Minor connector (C) Retentive arm (D) Reciprocal arm

REQUIREMENTS FOR CLASP ASSEMBLY DESIGN

1. Retention

It is the ability of clasp to resist dislodgement from the tooth in an occlusal direction away from the supporting tissue. The degree of retention possessed by the clasp is influenced by the amount of horizontal undercut engagement by the retentive tip and the resiliency of the clasp arm. **Clasp retention is a measure of resistance of the metal to deformation which is required for the clasp arm to escape from the undercut.**

2. Stabilization

It is the resistance to displacement in horizontal plane. Except the retentive tip all portion of clasp assembly contributes to stability.

3. Support

It is the property to resist gingival displacement. The occlusal (lingual/incisal) rest is the primary support unit.

4. Encirclement

The clasp should have a minimum three widespread point contact or 180 degree of abutment tooth encirclement to prevent slippage under forces.

5. Reciprocity

The retentive and reciprocal arm should be positioned on opposite side of tooth surface at the same horizontal plane. By doing so, the thrust exerted by the retentive arm as it flexes over the height of contour during insertion and removal is counterbalanced by the reciprocal arm.

6. Passivity

A clasp should not exert any pressure on tooth until it is moved by the prosthesis in function or when removed from the mouth.

7. Miscellaneous Considerations in Clasp Design

a. The buccolingual direction/depth of retentive undercut effects clasp retention.
b. Buccal or lingual, either of the two or both together can be used for clasp retention.
c. Molar compared to premolars needs less amount of undercut for retention. For a cast clasp;
   Molar = .0015″ undercut is required.
   Premolar = .0010″ undercut is required.
d. Clasping may be done for the reason of splinting adjacent teeth.
e. Clasp arm should be placed as low as permitted by survey line on the tooth for the reason of esthetic and leverage.

FACTORS OF CLASP RETENTION

Clasp retention is due to the resistance to deformation of clasp alloy, when dislodging forces are applied. Clasp retention is an effective product of two main factors.

1. Tooth Factors Which Includes

a. Depth of undercut.
b. Horizontal engagement of undercut.

2. Prosthesis Factors Which Includes

a. Clasp length and diameter.

b. Cross-sectional form of the clasp arm.

c. Material/alloy used

d. Angle of approach of clasp arm.

e. Position of the clasp in relation to fulcrum axis.

Depth of Undercut and Amount of Undercut Engagement

Both the vertical (depth) and the horizontal (amount) of undercut utilized below the survey line determines the retention. The lesser the vertical degree of engagement for a given or desired degree of horizontal undercut the more efficient will be the clasp. Thus, if the desirable undercut exists at 2 mm below the survey line going further down leads to greater stress on the abutment, failure and high chances of clasp deformation.

Clasp Length and Diameter

Longer the clasp arm greater will be the flexibility and more retention. Cast circumferential clasp arm with uniform taper from its origin to the retentive tip is more flexible than the bar clasp arm. Also, clasp made of gold alloys exhibits more flexibility over cobalt-chromium and give better retention. Greater the diameter of clasp arm lesser the flexibility for all other factors being equal.

Cross Sectional form of the Clasp Arm

Cast clasp are half round in cross section and hence can flex away or buccolingually only. Wrought wire clasp is all round in cross-section and can flex edgewise besides buccolingually thus providing better stress dissipiation.

Wrought wire clasp is the only circumferential clasp which can be used on an abutment tooth having undercut away from the distal extension base.

Material Used for Clasp Arm

Cobalt-chromium clasp are much stiffer than gold which are stiffer than the wrought alloy. Thus, for a given degree of undercut cobalt-chromium clasp can be made thinner for the required rigidity as compared to gold and wrought alloy which would require to be made bulkier.

Angle of Approach of the Clasp Arm
(Figs 2.23A to C)

The force required to displace a clasp arm from the tooth is dependent on the angle of approach of the tip to the plane of the undercut.

Gingivally approaching clasp arm exhibit tripping action or the push effect when dislodging forces are applied as compared to occlusally approaching clasp arm which exhibits pull action. Thus, by modifying the angle of approach of

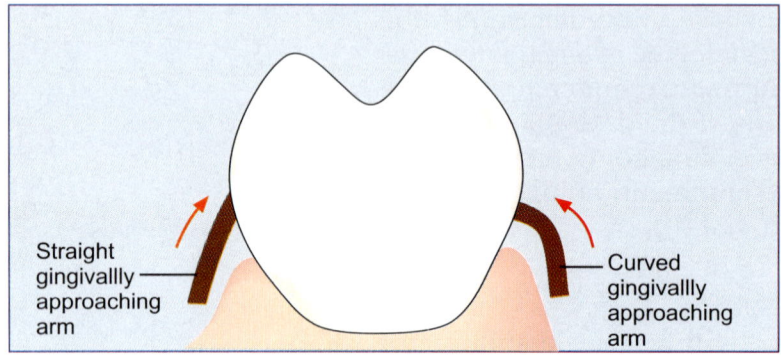

Fig. 2.23A

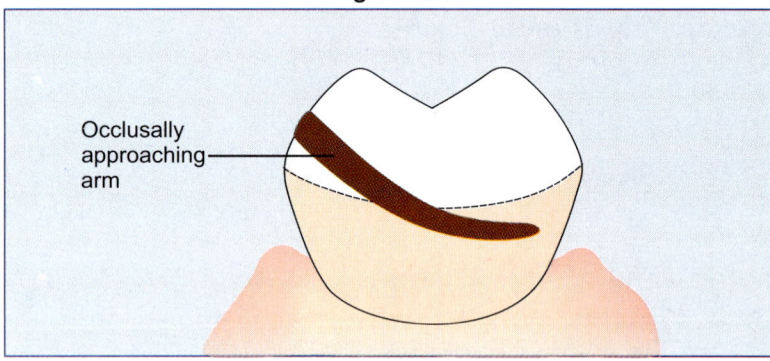

Fig. 2.23B

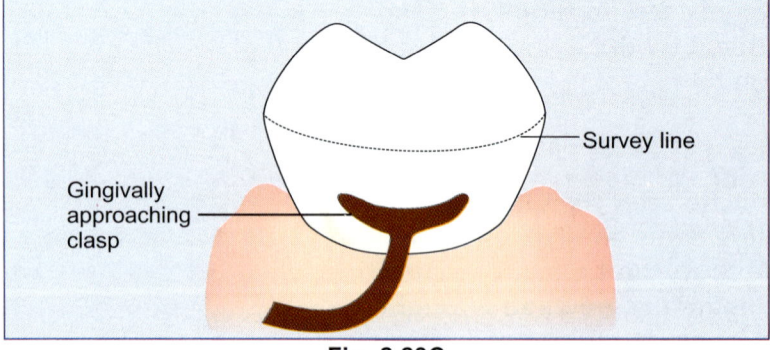

Fig. 2.23C

Figs 2.23A to C: The effect of increasing the angle of approach of the gingivally approaching arm by bending it near the contact surface, retention of clasp is increased. Gingivally approaching clasp are more retentive than occlusaly approaching

gingivally approaching arm, by a bend near the contacting surface of tooth, retention can be further enhanced.

Position of Clasp in Relation
to Fulcrum Axis

A fulcrum line is an imaginary line around which a distal extension denture is capable of rotating. The indirect retainer should be as far anterior as possible and the direct retainers should be as far away from the fulcrum axis for the best mechanical advantage.

CLASSIFICATION OF CLASP TYPES

Direct retainers or clasp assemblies can be classified as follows:

1. On the Basis of Construction

a. **The cast clasp** is fabricated by lost wax technique. It can be made of cobalt-chromium alloy, gold alloy or Titanium alloys.

b. **The wrought clasp** is made up of gold alloy wire, which is made from gold alloy by swaging and drawing through smaller die plates into desired shape and gauge. The wrought clasp, posses good resiliency but poor stabilizing properties.

c. **The combination clasp:** It consists of cast clasp assembly to which either gold alloy or Cobalt-Chromium alloy wrought retentive arm is added either by soldering or by embedding in the denture base. It combines the advantage of wrought clasp resiliency and cast clasp reciprocation and stabilizing properties. In addition, it has the capability to flex in all spatial planes thereby neutralizes the torsional forces and releases stress from the abutment tooth.

2. Clasp Classified on the Basis of Design

a. **The circumferential type** which approaches the undercut of the tooth above the survey line. The type of retention achieved is termed as PULL type and is also known as suprabulge clasp.

b. **The bar type:** The retentive terminal approaches the undercut from below the survey line. The bar clasp is also known as infrabulge or PUSH type.

3. Clasp which Provide Stress Control by Accommodating for Functional Prosthesis and Abutment Movement

a. Bar clasp
b. RPI
c. RPA
d. Combination clasp.

4. Clasp which do not Accommodate for Functional Movements.

Circumferential clasp.

DESCRIPTION OF TYPES OF CLASPS

Clasp will be basically discussed as:

1. Circumferential clasps and its types
2. Bar clasp, RPI, RPA
3. Combination clasp

Circumferential Clasp (Figs 2.24A and B)

i. Also known as Akers or class I clasp.
ii. It is used with tooth supported prosthesis where abutment teeth are healthy.
iii. It is primarily indicated when the retentive undercut is located on the buccal or lingual tooth surface away from the edentulous area.
iv. It provides excellent support, bilateral bracing and reciprocation.

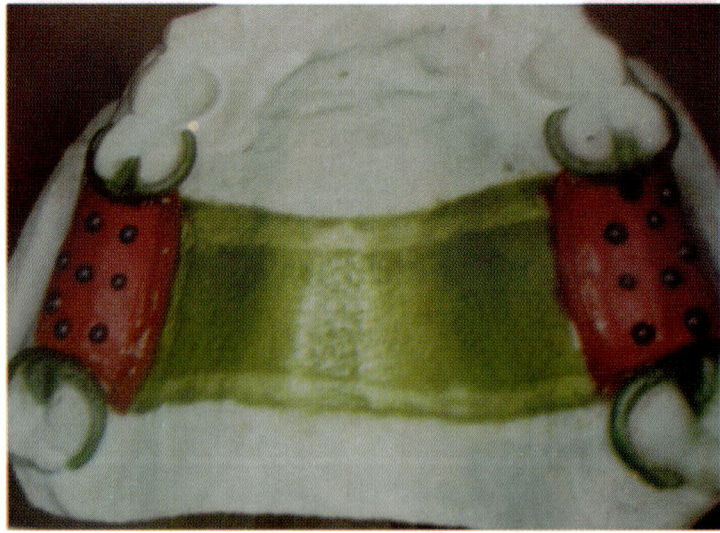

Fig. 2.24A

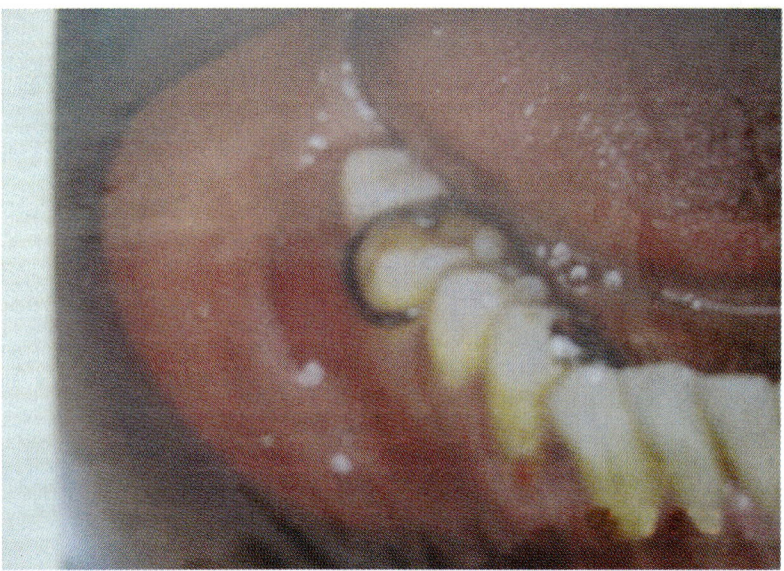

Fig. 2.24B

v. It requires 0.01 to 0.02 inch undercut for cast Cobalt-Chromium and cast gold alloy respectively.

vi. Its main disadvantage is poor esthetics, as it covers wider area of tooth structure.

vii. Increase risk of caries to abutment tooth.

- *Ring Clasp* **(Fig. 2.25)**

i. The ring clasp is used when a proximal undercut cannot be approached by other means as in bucally inclined maxillary molars and lingually inclined mandibular molars.

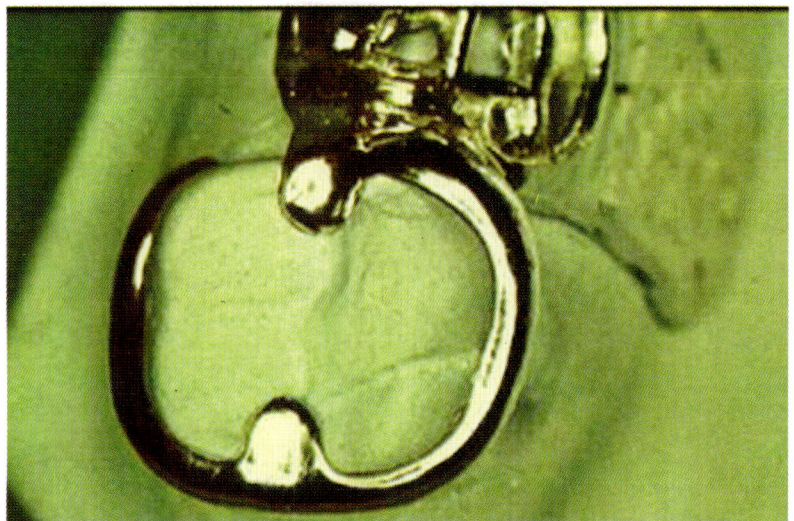

Fig. 2.25: Ring clasp

ii. A ring clasp originates from one proximal surface (minor connector) encircles the tooth completely to engage an undercut directly below the rest seat at the point of origin.

iii. A ring clasp should be well supported by accessory minor connector and auxilliary rest.

iv. It covers wide area of tooth surface.

- *Embrasure Clasp* **(Fig. 2.26)**

    i. Embrasure clasp are indicated in Kennedy's Class II, unilateral distal extension removable partial dentures where there are no modification spaces.

    ii. It provides cross-arch bracing support and retention.

    iii. It uses transocclusal rest, two reciprocal arm and two retentive arm on two adjoining teeth on the side opposite to edentulous area.

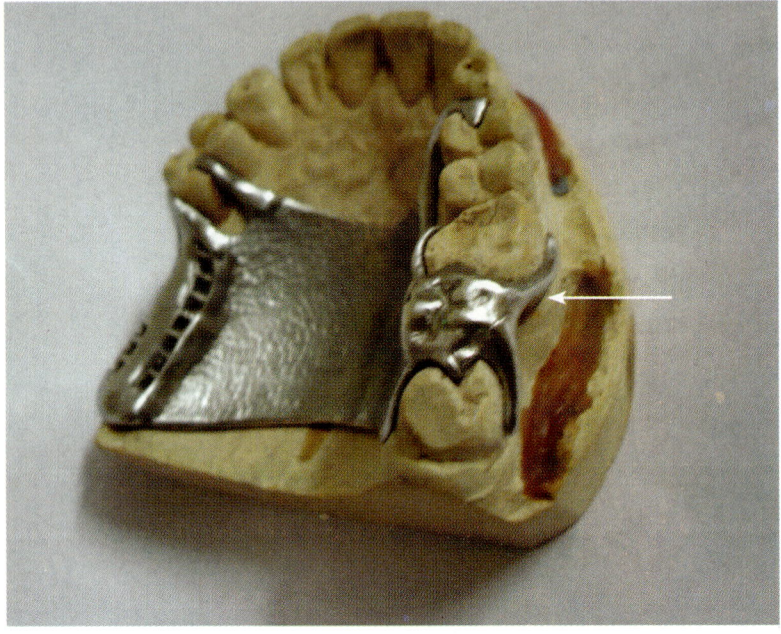

Fig. 2.26: Embrasure clasp

    iv. Retention and reciprocation can be reversed on both teeth or on either tooth depending upon the contours and undercut.

- *Multiple Clasp* **(Fig. 2.27)**

    i. It consist of two opposing circumferential clasp joined at the terminal end of the two reciprocal arm.

ii. It can be used in lieu of embrasure clasp, when multiple clasping for additional retention and stability is required as in long span unilateral edentulous arches replacing entire half arch.

- *Half and Half Clasp*
   i. It consist of facial half and a lingual half originating from separate minor connectors.
  ii. The facial portion is the facial half of a circumferential clasp.
 iii. The lingual portion originates from a minor connector and rest in the mesial and lingual embrasure of the abutment tooth.
  iv. It is indicated on a pier abutment or on unilateral partial denture design.

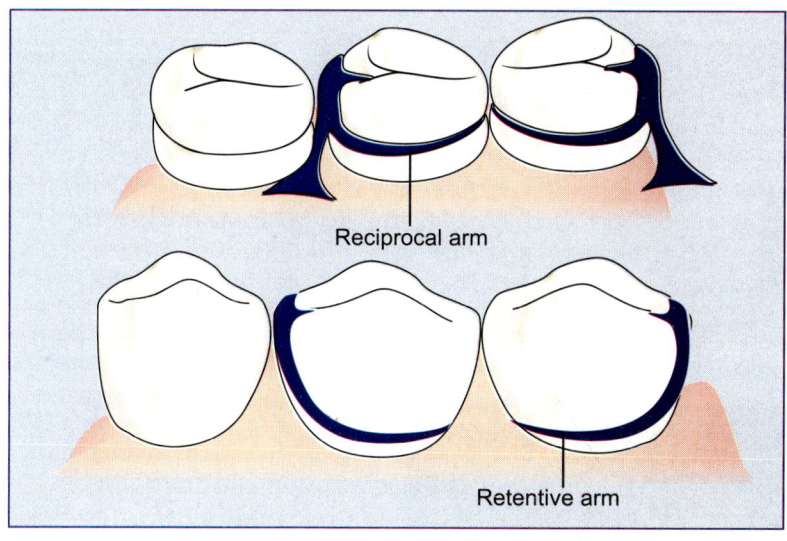

Reciprocal arm

Retentive arm

Fig. 2.27: Multiple clasp

- *Reverse Action Clasp (Fig. 2.28)*
   i. Also known as hairpin clasp
  ii. It engages a proximal undercut directly below the point of origin from occlusal direction.
 iii. It is used in lieu of ring clasp or bar clasp when tissue undercuts, high tissue attachments or lingual inclination of abutment teeth prevents their usage.
  iv. It covers wide tooth surface and is unesthetic.

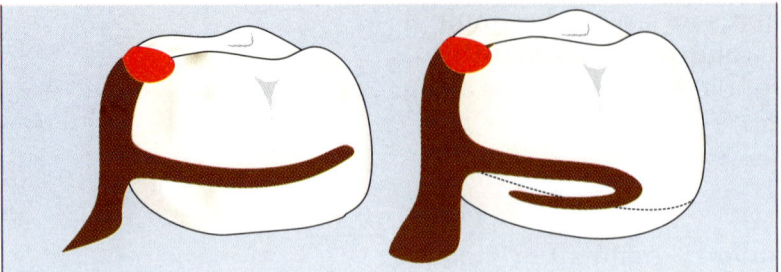

Fig. 2.28: Reverse action / Hair pin clasp

Bar Clasp (Figs 2.29A and B)

i. Also known as infrabulge or Roach clasp. They are classified by the shape of their retentive terminus.

ii. Bar clasp originates from the denture base or the metal framework and approaches the undercut from the gingival direction. The retentive terminus takes the shape of Y, T, modified T or I-bar.

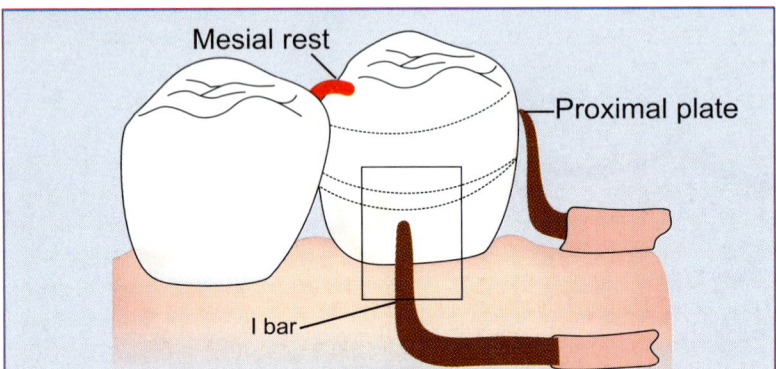

Fig. 2.29A

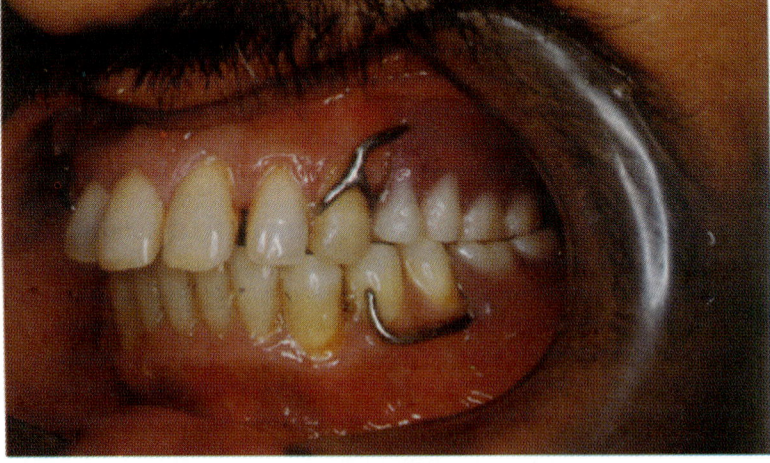

Fig. 2.29B

Figs 2.29A and B: Bar clasp

iii. Bar clasp provides push type of retention and since, they cover smaller area of tooth surface they are more esthetic.

iv. Bar clasp are used when the retentive undercut is located on the middle or on the buccal or lingual surface of the tooth adjacent to the edentulous area.

v. Bar clasp consist of mesial rest, proximal plate and approach arm with retentive terminus.

vi. The proximal plate contacts the guiding plane of the abutment tooth from just below the marginal ridge and extend gingivally to the junction of middle and gingival third.
Proximal plate is 1 mm thick and should contact approximately two thirds of the buccolingual width of the abutment tooth and extends to the lingual axial line angle to provide for bracing.

vii. Modified T-bar is used instead of T-bar clasp on maxillary canines and premolars for reason of esthetics.

- *RPI Clasp*

Rest, proximal plate and I-bar clasp (Fig. 2.30).

i. Coined by **Krol** in 1973 (Figs 2.31A and B).

ii. It consists of a mesio-occlusal rest with the minor connector placed in the mesio-lingual embrasure but not contacting the adjacent tooth.

iii. Distal guiding plane extending from the marginal ridge to the junction of middle and gingival thirds of abutment tooth and is contacted by the proximal plate.

iv. I-bar: located in the gingival third in 0.01″ undercut and no more than 2 mm of its tip should contact the abutment.

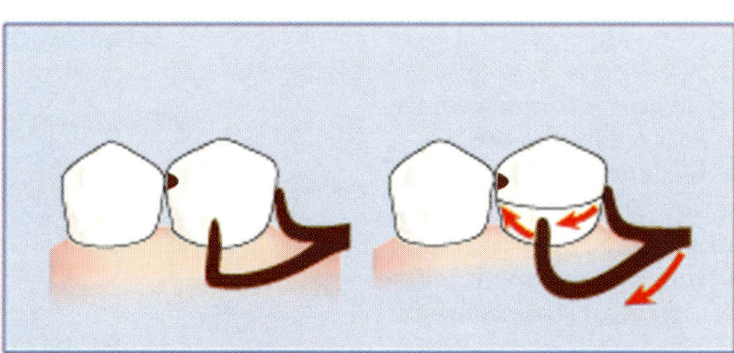

Fig. 2.30: RPI clasp design

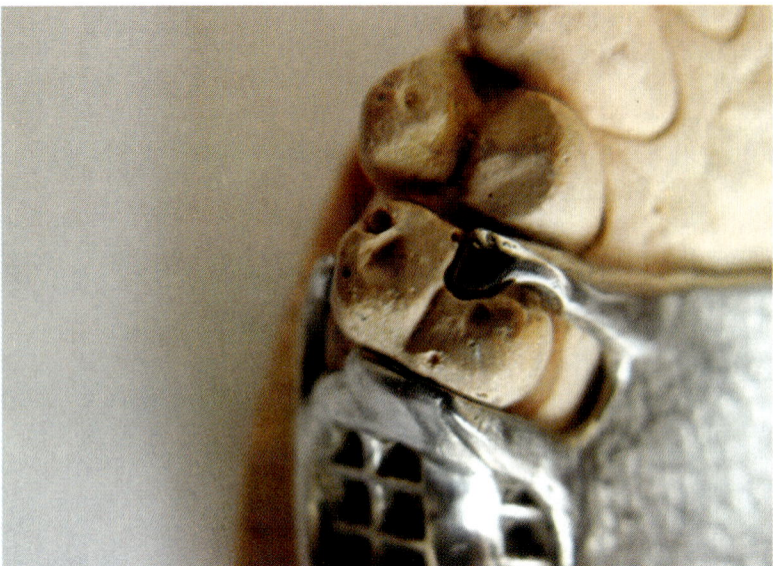

Fig. 2.31A

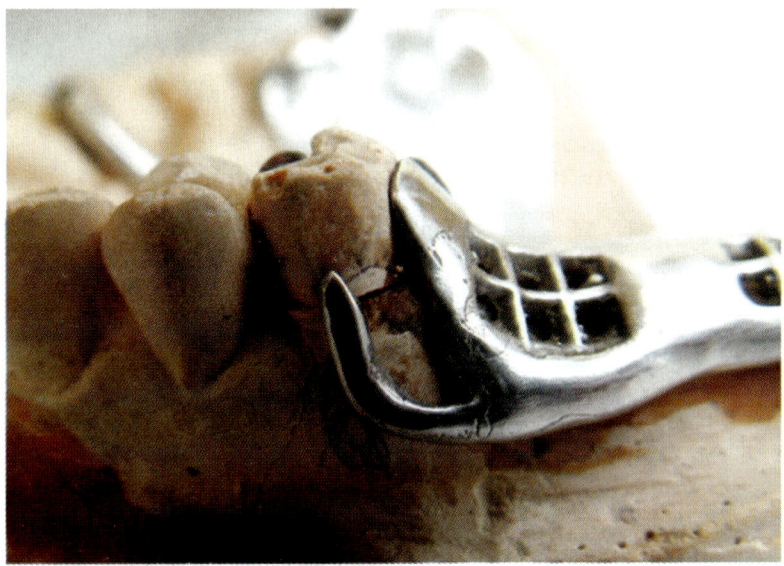

Fig. 2.31B

Figs 2.31A and B: Showing RPI clasp asembly. It consists of mesial occlusal rest, proximal plate contacting guide plane and I- bar clasp

v. Occlusal rest minor connector and proximal plate provides clasp reciprocation and encirclement.

vi. RPI is a self releasing clasp. As the denture base is placed under function, rotation occurs around the mesial occlusal rests bilaterally. Simultaneously, the proximal plates and I bars disengages from the abutment teeth thereby preventing transfer of harmful stresses to the abutment tooth.

- *RPA Clasp*

  i. It consist of mesioocclusal rest and proximal plate contacting the tooth surface adjacent to the edentulous base area extending from the marginal ridge to the junction of middle and gingival third of the abutment tooth.

  ii. The retentive component is a modified circumferential clasp in which the circumferential arm arises from the proximal plate adjacent to the edentulous base area.

  iii. It is indicated with distal extension removable partial denture when the retentive undercut is located on the facial surface away from the edentulous area.

3. Combination Clasp

Described earlier in the text

Blatterfeins Classificafion of Survey Lines (Figs 2.32A to C)

Survey line delineates the height of contour of the tooth, Blatterfein described that abutment tooth could be divided into two halves by a vertical line through the long axis of the tooth. He termed the two halves as the near zone (towards the saddle) and far zone (away from the saddle).

According to Blatterfein, there are four types of survey lines possible passing through the buccal or lingual surface of abutment tooth. The type of survey line will influence the selection of clasp types for that particular tooth.

1. The Medium Survey Line

It appear on the buccal or lingual surface of the tooth, approximately equidistant from the occlusal and gingival margin in the near zone and slightly closer to the gingival margin in the far zone.

Choice of Clasp

a.**Occlusaly approaching:** Circumferential clasp
b.**Gingivally approaching:** Bar clasp.

2. The Diagonal Survey Line

This survey line lies nearer the occlusal surface than the gingival margin in the near zone of the tooth but in the far zone it is closer to the gingival margin.

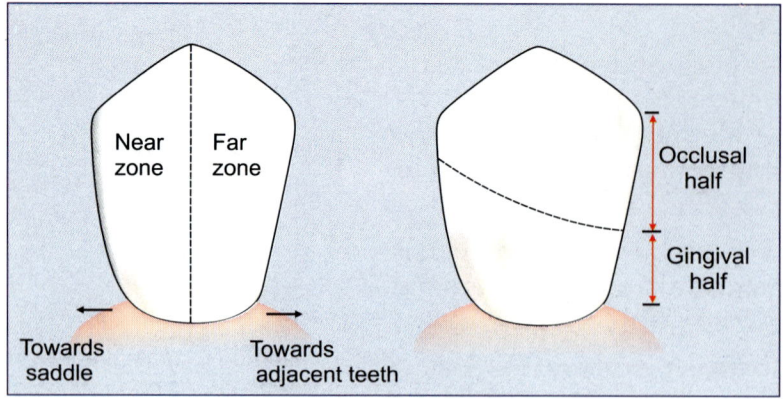

Fig. 2.32A: Medium

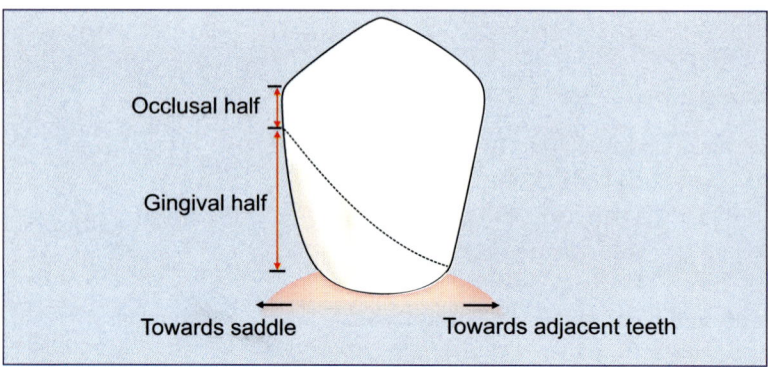

Fig. 2.32B: Diagnoal

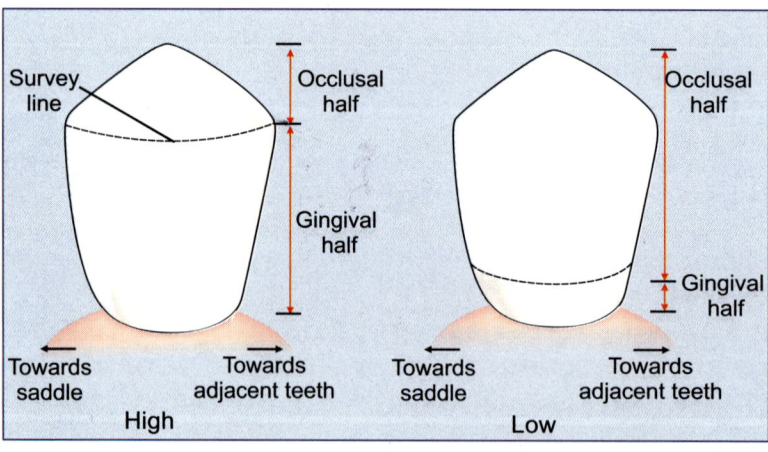

Fig. 2.32C: High and Low

Figs 2.32A to C: Blatterfein's Classification of survey line as (A) Medium (B) Diagonal (C) High and Low

Choice of Clasp

a. **Occlusal approaching:** Reverse action clasp/ring clasp.
b. **Gingivally approaching:** L or T-shaped bar clasp.

3. High Survey Line

This survey line appears much nearer to the occlusal than the gingival of the abutment tooth in both near and far zone.

The choice of clasp is wrought wire clasp. Gingivally approaching clasp are of little use.

4. Low Survey Line

The survey line lies low on the buccal or lingual aspect of a tooth. Tooth surface with low survey line cannot receive a retentive arm but may receive a reciprocal arm. However following options could be considered for the tooth with low survey line.

a. **Using the proximal undercut:** De Van clasp.
b. **Using the extended arm clasp:** Where in the adjacent tooth is also included in the coverage of clasp assembly.
c. Crowning the tooth and developing appropriate contours for clasping.

CLASP DESIGN: POINTS TO REMEMBER

1. A clasp should always be supported by rest.
2. A molar ring clasp should have occlusal rests mesially and distally.
3. A molar ring clasp, which engages lingual undercut should have a buccal strengthening arm.
4. Retentive clasps can be used to provide indirect support for a distal extension saddle by being placed on the opposite side of the support axis from the saddle.
5. A wrought wire clasp should be attached to a saddle, not to exposed parts of the metal framework.
6. An occlusally approaching clasp should not approach closer than 1 mm to the gingival margin.
7. A retentive occlusally approaching clasp should run from the side of the tooth with the least undercut to the side with the greatest undercut.
8. 0.25 mm of undercut is required for retentive clasp when done in Co-Cr alloy.

9. If the retentive undercut is less than 0.25 mm then either dimpling or composite resin be added to the tooth to create the required amount of undercut.

10. The retentive arm should be minimum 15 mm in length and taper gradually from its point of origin when made in Co-Cr alloy.

11. Occlusally approaching retentive clasp should be restricted to molars when made in Co-Cr alloy. For premolars wrought wire is preferred.

12. A retentive clasp arm should engage 0.5 mm of undercut if it is constructed in wrought wire.

13. A retentive clasp should be at least 7 mm in length if it is constructed in wrought wire.

14. Retentive clasps should usually be placed buccally on upper teeth and lingually on lower molars. For premolars and canines retentive clasps are usually placed buccally.

15. Buccal or lingual retention on one side of the arch should be opposed by Buccal or lingual retention on the other side of the arch.

16. Clasp assembly should encircle the tooth by more than 180 degrees.

17. Reciprocation arm should be located diametrically opposite the retentive clasp tip and at the level of middle of middle third.

18. Guide plate instead of reciprocal arm can be used for providing reciprocation.

19. Gingivally approaching clasps are contraindicated where the buccal sulcus is less than 4 mm in depth or more than 1 mm undercut.

20. RPI system can be used on premolar abutment for distal extension bases. The other choices are wrought wire clasp and RPA clasp.

21. For all the Kennedy classes the use of minimum two clasps is advantageous because two clasp usually provide sufficient retention and keeps the design simple. Also, two clasp forms a clasp axis that can be positioned to bisect the denture and allows indirect retention to be obtained.

22. Bounded saddles should have a clasp at least at one end.

23. A Kennedy Class IV should have retentive clasp on the first molars if there is a suitable undercut present.

MULTIPLE CHOICE QUESTIONS

1. **Which of the following clasp system are not indicated for extension base partial dentures?**
   A. Cast Circumferential clasp
   B. Bar clasp
   C. Mesial back action clasp
   D. Cast combination clasp.

2. **RPI Bar concept is a modified "Kratochvil" concept which of the following is not true for RPI concept?**
   A. Modified by Krol
   B. Minimizes stress on abutment
   C. Consist of mesial rest, proximal plate
   D. I-bar moves buccally under masticatory load.

3. **Which of the following regarding the design of RPI clasp is not true?**
   A. Mesio-occlusal rest, with minor connector not contacting adjacent tooth.
   B. Proximal plate at the junction of middle and cervical third proximally.
   C. Guide plane prepared up to the junction of occlusal and middle one third on distal surface.
   D. I-bar located in 0.01 inch undercut and at the greatest mesio distal prominence.

4. **Which of the following is not an advantage of the RPI clasp system?**
   A. Disengagement of abutment both by clasp and proximal plate under function.
   B . Adequate reciprocation from mesial minor connector and proximal plate.
   C. Esthetic and low caries incidence.
   D. Mesial rest provides pump handle effect on the distal abutment.

5. **Location of mesial rest as compared to distal in extension base partial dentures is advantageous because of:**
   A. Mesial rest maintains contacts with anterior teeth.
   B. Elimination of class I leverages.
   C. More vertical loading of residual ridge.
   D. All of the above.

6. **Which of the following is not a contraindication for RPI clasp?**
   A. Insufficient depth of vestibule
   B. Abnormal inclination of abutment teeth
   C. Presence of only distobuccal undercut
   D. Use of linguoplate major connector on abutment tooth
   E. Unilateral distal extension base

7. **RPA clasp is indicated when/for?**
   A. Tooth supported partial dentures
   B. T-bar is contraindicated
   C. Distobuccal undercut is present
   D. Mid-buccal undercut is present

8. **Bar clasp are more retentive than circumferential clasp:**

   True/False

9. **Bar type clasp assembly is indicated:**
   A. When the undercut is away from edentulous area
   B. Mid buccal undercut
   C. Low survey line
   D. Undercut adjacent to edentulous area.

10. **Most common cause of failure of bar clasp is:**
    A. Less reciprocation
    B. Soft tissue undercuts
    C. Poor retention
    D. Improper design of clasp assembly

11. **In a distal extension situation when a RPI bar clasp assembly is employed the contact of proximal plate with the prepared guide plane is decided by all of the following *except*:**
    A. Length of the edentulous span
    B. Quality and quantity of ridge
    C. Periodontal health of the abutment
    D. Simplicity of design
    E. Location of the undercut

12. **Combination clasp acts as a stress release clasp when used in distal extension situations. The main reason to use it over other clasp assembly are:**
    A. When the undercut is away from edentulous side
    B. When the distal abutment is weak
    C. When pier abutment is present
    D. None of the above

NOTES

13. **For the same amount of undercut which of the following clasp will be more flexible?**
    A. 0.7 inch bar clasp
    B. 0.7 inch circumferential clasp
    C. 0.7 inch wrought wire clasp
    D. Equal flexibility

14. **Half round form of cast clasp permit flexing in what direction:**
    A. Occlus gingival
    B. Labio lingual
    C. Mesio distal
    D. Permit 360 degree movement

15. **Reciprocal arm should contact the abutment slightly before the retentive arm. Which of the following is function of reciprocal arm:**
    A. Resist tooth movement due to retentive arm deformation
    B. Denture stabilization and cross arch stability
    C. Indirect retention
    D. All of the above

16. **Direct retainers provide mechanical retention by all means as below *except*:**

    A. Friction
    B. Engaging undercut
    C. Engaging depression/dimpling
    D. Active tooth contact

17. **Intracoronal retainer provides retention by:**
    A. Abrasion
    B. Frictional contact
    C. Parallel tooth walls
    D. Precision labial retentive arm

18. **Extracoronal clasp retention is by:**
    A. Frictional resistance
    B. Flexible resistance arm
    C. Resistance of alloy to deformation
    D. All of the above

19. **Function of clasp arm is all *except*:**
    A. Support
    B. Stabilization
    C. Reciprocation
    D. Retention

NOTES

20. **Part of direct retainer assembly which lies below the high of contour is?**
    A. Reciprocal arm
    B. Shoulder
    C. Retentive tip
    D. Middle portion of retentive arm along with the tip

21. **The part of direct retainer which connects retentive tip to body of clasp is:**
    A. Shoulder
    B. Truss arm
    C. Tang
    D. Reciprocal arm

22. **Greater the angle of cervical convergence on the abutment tooth placement of retentive tip would be:**
    A. Near the survey line
    B. More gingivally into the undercut
    C. Midway into the undercut
    D. More horizontally located into the undercut

23. **Blatterfein classified clasp line as:**
    A. High and low
    B. Medium
    C. Diagonal
    D. All of the above

24. **Bar clasp give retention by:**
    A. Push action
    B. Pull action
    C. Whiplash effect
    D. None of the above

25. **Amount of undercut required for wrought wire clasp:**
    A. .01 inch
    B. .015 inch
    C. .020 inch
    D. .025 inch

26. **The most important factor in clasp designing is:**
    A. Location of undercut
    B. Height of undercut
    C. Width of undercut
    D. Number of undercuts

27. **For clasp retention to be effective, retentive undercut should be present:**
    A. Parallel to path of placement
    B. Parallel to path of displacement
    C. Parallel to path of removal
    D. None of the above

28. **Which of the following clasp involves inter-proximal undercut?**
    A. Devan
    B. Reverse action
    C. Hairpin
    D. I-bar

29. **Embrasure clasps are best used for:**
    D. Kennedy Cl II situation
    B. Kennedy's Cl I situation
    C. Kennedy's Cl III modification I
    D. All of the above

30. **The main indication for using hairpin clasp is:**
    A. When undercut exists below the point of origin
    B. When bar type retentive arm is contraindicated
    C. Esthetics are objectionable
    D. All of the above

ANSWERS

1 C

2 D RPI consists of three separate units connected to each other only through the framework. It consists of occlusal rest located mesially, I-bar clasp placed midbucally on the abutment and proximal plate contacting the distal and distolingual surfaces of the abutment adjacent to the edentulous space.

3 B The superior edge of the proximal plate is located at the bottom of the prepared guide plane which should be at the junction of the occlusal one third and middle one third of the tooth.

4 D

5 D Placement of the occlusal rest mesial to the point of contact of the retentive bearing changes the forces on the tooth from class 1 to class 2 types of lever action. In class 2, the retentive arm is located posterior to the fulcrum than the rest.

6 E

7 B RPA clasp may be used in place of RPI clasp when there is insufficient depth of the buccal vestibule or when buccal tissue undercut is too great. It is same as RPI except that in place of 1-bar, there is a circumferential Akers arm arising from the proximal plate.

8 True

Due to longer bar type clasp arms, the tripping action (gingivally approaching) and location of undercut (adjacent to the edentulous area) these clasp are more retentive.

9 D

10 D

11 D, E

12 B Combination clasp consists of cast reciprocal arm and a wrought wire (18 or 19 gauge PDP round wire) retentive arm.

Advantage: flexibility, adjustability, appearance.

Disadvantage: extra laboratory steps in fabrication, easily distorted on mishandling and in function.

Combination clasp are indicated on distal extension abutments which are weak and undercut exists away from edentulous site and cannot be approached by gingivally approaching arm.

13 C For the same length of clasp wrought wire would be more flexible as it is all round and will flex 360 in all spatial planes. Whereas, for the same length circumferential clasp would be more retentive as compared to bar clasp because, bar clasp half-round form lies in several planes from its point of origin, which prevents its flexibility from being proportional to its total length.

14 B Cast clasp can flex away from tooth but edgewise flexing is limited.

15 D   Reciprocal arm can also act as an indirect retainer when placed on suprabulge area of an abutment tooth lying anterior to the fulcrum line.

16 D
17 B
18 C
19 A
20 D
21 A
22 A
23 D
24 A
25 C
26 A
27 B
28 A
29 A
30 A

INDIRECT RETAINERS

Definition: Indirect retainer is that component of a removable partial denture which resists rotational movement of the distal extension base away from the basal seat by supporting the framework opposite to the fulcrum axis and indirectly activating the direct retainers to prevent denture dislodgement (Fig. 2.33).

> Indirect retainer is an occlusal, incisal or cingulum rest having proper contact in well prepared rest seat.

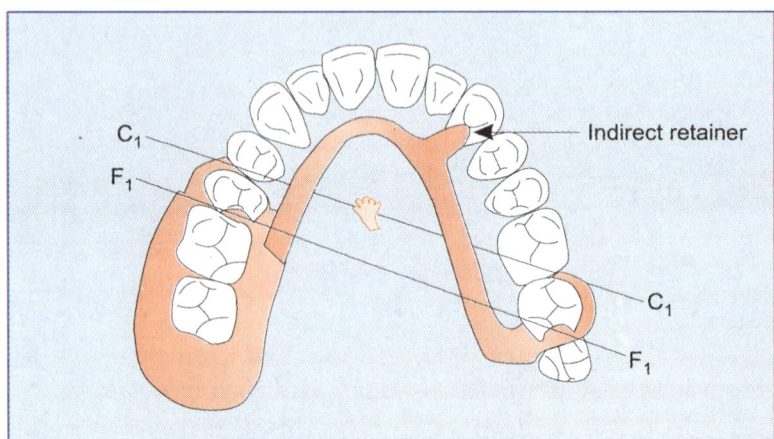

Fig. 2.33: Showing fulcrum line (F_1–F_1) and clasp line (C_1–C_1)

> **Fulcrum line (1916, Prothero)** is an imaginary axis passing through the most posterior abutment on either side of the arch around which the distal extension denture will rotate as the base move away from the residual ridge.

Rationale for Indirect Retention

Extension based partial dentures which are both tooth and tissue supported (Kennedy's Class I, Class II, long span Class IV) unlike tooth supported dentures (Kennedy's Class III, short span Class IV) can move around fulcrum line either away or towards the basal seat.

An extension base denture, having a stress release clasp on distal abutment, will rotate towards and away from the basal seat around a fulcrum point which is in the form of a primary rest on the distal abutment. As the denture rotates around the fulcrum away from the basal seat, the major connector opposite to the fulcrum line and away from the extension base would then move inferiorly, causing impingement and injuring the soft tissue underneath (Fig. 2.34).

This inferior movement of the extension based Removable Partial denture can be best prevented by placing auxilliary or secondary rests in the well prepared rest seat anterior/ opposite to the fulcrum line. This also shifts the fulcrum anterior and there by activates the direct retainers to grip the abutment and prevent displacement of the denture (Fig. 2.35).

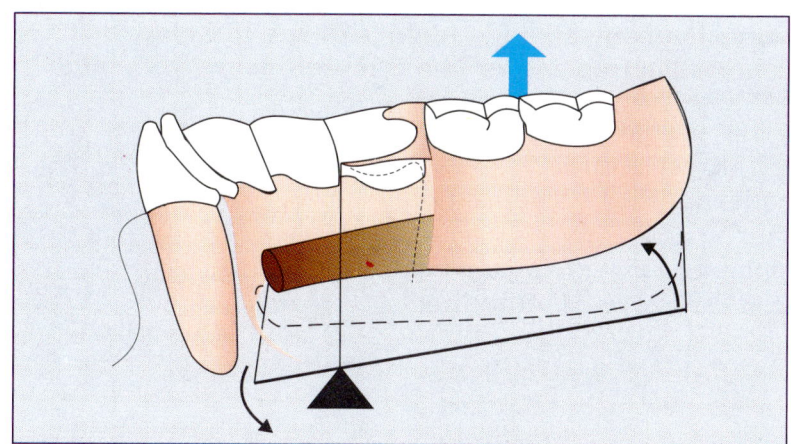

Fig. 2.34: Need for indirect retention. As the dislodging forces (arrow) due to forces of gravity, mastication and stickiness of food tries to lift the distal extension prosthesis away from the saddle, the denture rotates around the occlusal rest (primary abutment) and the major connector anteriorly moves down inferiorly stripping the lingual gingiva. In this whole process the clasp tip of the primary abutments gets activated and deformed

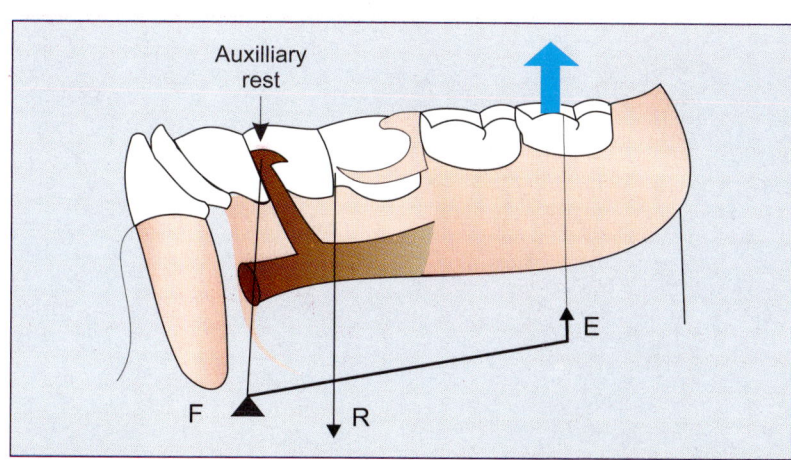

Fig. 2.35: Rationale for indirect retainer. The indirect retainer concept consist of preventing the displacement of a free end saddle by creating a lever system (Class III). An indirect retainer for a free end saddle is a supporting element (Auxillary rest) on the other side of a line joining a clasp axis. The anterior placement of rest (auxilliary rest) will now prevent gingival displacement of the major connector anteriorly and activate the direct retainer to resist displacement

Guidelines for Indirect Retainer Functioning (Fig. 2.36)

i. Identification and location of fulcrum axis should be done around which the rotational movement will occur.
ii. Indirect Retainer positioning:
   • Should be placed perpendicular to the fulcrum line
   • Should be as far away (and opposite) to the fulcrum line as possible
   • Should be placed in well prepared rest seats on teeth capable of best providing support.
   • Canines and premolars both in maxillae and mandible are preferred over incisors.
iii. All minor connectors joining the indirect retainer to the major connectors should be rigid.

Functions of Indirect Retainer

i. Prevents movement of prosthesis away from basal seat in extension based removable partial denture.
ii. Minor connector joining indirect retainer to major connector is rigid and provides additional stabilization of prosthesis.
iii. Major connector like linguoplate or Kennedy's bar when supported by auxilliary rest can serve as an indirect retainer.
iv. Indirect retainer may provide the first visual indication for the need to reline an extension based partial denture.
   The indirect retainer always works at mechanical disadvantage. By incorporating indirect ratainer in a free end situation, the resistance to effort arm is increased.

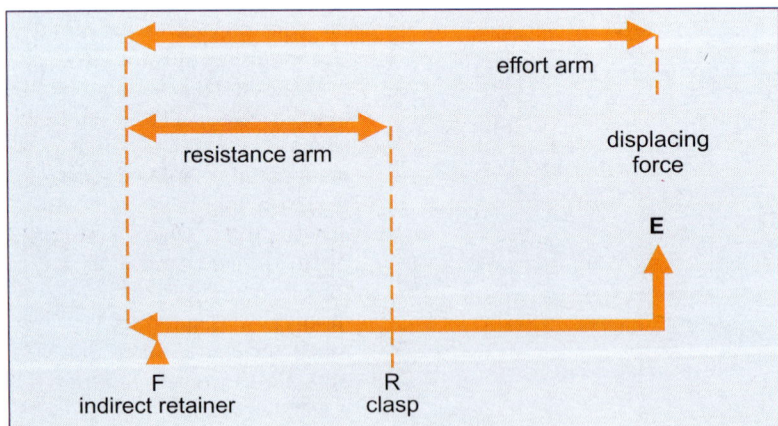

effort arm

displacing force

E

resistance arm

F
indirect retainer

R
clasp

Fig. 2.36: The concept of location of indirect retainer.

$$\text{Mechanical disadvantage} = \frac{\text{resistance arm}}{\text{effort arm}}$$

$$= \frac{\text{distance between clasp and indirect retainer}}{\text{distance between point of effort and indirect retainer}}$$

Forms of Indirect Retainer (Table 2.8)

Table 2.8: Forms of indirect return to retainer	
Occlusal Rest	• Secondary or auxilliary rest acts as an indirect retainer • Most commonly on the mesial marginal ridge of first premolars in class I situation • Auxilliary occlusal rest should be placed in well formed rest seat
Canine Rest	Cingulum of canine is used for placing indirect retainer when mesial marginal ridge of first premolar is close to the fulcrum axis
Canine extension	Finger extension on canine from occlusal rest on first premolar where first premolar rest is the primary rest and canine extension acts as indirect retention
Linguo-plate	Whenever linguoplate or continuous bars are supported by auxilliary/ occlusal/canine rest at either ends it serves as indirect retainer
Modifica-tion area	In Kennedy Class II mod 1,the anterior abutment on the tooth bounded side can receive occlusal rest and serve as indirect retainer
Rugae	In maxillary arch rugae when covered by maxillary major connector serves to provide indirect retention as in horse shoe major connector

MULTIPLE CHOICE QUESTIONS

1. **Which of the following component act as a third point of reference while positioning the partial denture framework on the teeth?**
   A. Occlusal rest
   B. Direct retainer
   C. Indirect retainer
   D. Major connector

2. **For indirect retainer to be most effective the clasp must be placed:**
   A. Between the saddle and proximal plate
   B. Anterior to fulcrum line
   C. Posterior to the fulcrum line
   D. Near the major connector

3. **Function of indirect retainer is to:**
   A. Provide retention
   B. Prevent displacement
   C. Provides support primarily
   D. Prevent movement away from the edentulous ridge

4. **Fulcrum line/Axis:**
   A. Passes through the suprabulge component of clasp located on primary abutment.
   B. Same as clasp axis
   C. Coined by BalkWill
   D. Passes through the retentive portion of clasp assembly on primary abutment.

5. **Indirect retainer acts mainly to:**
   A. Prevent settling of denture
   B. Provide retention, stability and support
   C. Prevents lingual tooth migration
   D. Activates direct retainers during displacement

6. **Indirect retainer form is/or consists of:**
   A. Primary rest
   B. Rest and proximal plate
   C. Primarily auxilliary rest
   D. None of the above

7. **Location of indirect retainer should be:**
   A. Closer to fulcrum line
   B. Anterior and forward to fulcrum line

C. Perpendicular to fulcrum line

D. In a well formed rest seat on a healthy abutment.

8. **Which of the following can be used as indirect retainer?**
   A. Incisal rest
   B. Linguoplate
   C. Modification areas
   D. Rugae support
   E. All of the above

9. **Which of the following situations do not require indirect retention?**
   A. Kennedy's Cl I, Cl II
   B. Kennedy's Cl III mod I
   C. Long span Cl IV
   D. Cl III with poor abutment support

10. **Bilaterally placed indirect retainers in mandibular Kennedy's situation are used for:**
    A. Increased effectiveness of direct retainers
    B. Support major connector
    C. Compensates for close location of indirect retainer to fulcrum line
    D. Auxilliary function only

11. **Function of distal extension partial denture is affected by residual ridge resorption. Which of the following is true regarding alveolar resorption?**
    A. Chronic and continuous in nature
    B. Maximum reduction upto 2 years
    C. Accelerated by denture wearing immediately after extraction
    D. All of the above
    E. None of the above

12. **Combination syndrome given by Kelly, occurs due to:**
    A. Maxillary partial denture
    B. Maxillary and mandibular complete denture
    C. Mandibular anteriors against maxillary complete denture
    D. None of the above

13. **Which of the following is not a feature of combination syndrome?**
    A. RRR in anterior mandible
    B. Downgrowth of maxillary tuberosity

C. Papillary hyperplasia over hard palate

D. Extrusion of mandibular anterior teeth

14. **The first visual indication of a distal extension requiring relining is:**
    A. Lifting up of indirect retainers
    B. Loss of occlusal contact
    C. Decrease in vertical dimension
    D. Commissure at the corner of the mouth

15. **The need to reline a extension base partial denture is determined by which of the following technique:**
    A. Alginate wash
    B. Looseness of direct retainer
    C. Tissue ward movement of major connector
    D. All of the above

16. **Rebasing of partial denture base is indicated for all of the following reasons** *except*:
    A. Denture base porosity
    B. Fractured and unesthetic denture base
    C. Inadequate denture base extension
    D. Residual ridge reduction only

17. **Which of the following impression material are least suited for making relining impression?**
    A. Impression plaster
    B. Free flowing ZOE
    C. Mouth temperature waxes
    D. Tissue conditioning material

18. **Which of the following is not a reason for relining of partial denture?**
    A. Excessive occlusal wear
    B. Lifting of indirect retainer
    C. Rotation of denture around fulcrum axis
    D. Unesthetic denture base

19. **A 34-year old patient wearing 8 week old mandibular bilateral distal extension RPD exhibits occlusal wear. What would be the treatment for same?**
    A. Reline
    B. Rebase
    C. Occlusal reconstruction
    D. Remake

20. **Which of the following is not the purpose of indirect retainer?**
    A. Support major connector
    B. Increased effectiveness of clasp
    C. Serves as primary rest
    D. Stabilization

ANSWERS

1 C Indirect retainer helps in positioning the framework on the teeth during relining procedure and during altered cast impression for distal extension base RPD.

2 C Further the clasp placed towards the saddle area more will be the mechanical advantage. Indirect retainer should be placed as far anterior/away from the saddle as possible.

3 D

4 A

5 D

6 C Indirect retainer is primarily auxilliary or secondary rest and its supporting minor connector. The proximal plate, adjacent to the edentulous area may also provide indirect retention.

7 B,D

8 E

9 B

10 B

11 D

12 C Kelly's/combination syndrome occurs in patient with mandibular bilateral distal extension opposing maxillary complete denture.

13 A

14 A

15 A A thin mix of alginate material may be applied to the fitting surface of the denture base for determining the amount of ridge reduction. If at least 2 mm of alginate is present under the denture base it indicates a need for relining or rebasing.

16 D Relining involves adding new denture base material to the existing resin, to make up for the loss of tissue contact caused by alveolar ridge resorption.

Rebasing is a laboratory technique where the bulk of the denture base is removed and replaced using new resin.

17 D Tissue conditioners can be used for reline impressions but can easily distort soft tissues.

18 A,D Rebasing is indicated for the following:
- Excessive occlusal wear
- Unesthetic denture base
- Improper denture base extension
- Loss of vertical dimension of occlusion

19 C Re-establishment of occlusal surface in harder material, e.g. (metal occlusal).

20 C They act as auxilliary or secondary rest.

DENTURE TEETH AND DENTURE BASE CONSIDERATIONS

Prosthetic teeth for removable partial denture should be pleasing in appearance, adaptable to any edentulous space, easily attach to the prosthesis, should be unbreakable and resistant to wear. They can be made up in variety of material:

 i. Cross linked acrylic resin
 ii. Composite resin
 iii. Metal
 iv. Porcelain

Most common material used for prosthetic teeth is either cross linked acrylic resin or porcelain. (Table 2.9)

Table 2.9: Differences between acrylic resin or porcelain teeth	
Acrylic teeth	*Porcelain teeth*
Strong in thin sections, can be recontoured to fit in limited interridge space	Can not be altered, weak in thin section
Percolation: Seepage of fluid around the neck of teeth and denture base is eliminated due to chemical bonding	Percolation around porcelain teeth occurs due to polymerization shrinkage of methylmethacrylate resin
Resistance to wear is low hence it is kinder to opposing enamel	Porcelain teeth are harder. They abrade opposing enamel and transfers greater load to the residual alveolar ridge.
Acrylic teeth are prone to staining	Porcelain is impervious to staining
Acrylic teeth are less noisy	Porcelain teeth are more prone to produce clicking noise, in the patient who do not possess good neuro muscular control.
They are chemically bonded to denture bases	Porcelain teeth are mechanically held through diatoric holes.
Dentures with acrylic teeth are difficult to rebase	Denture with porcelain teeth are easier to rebase

PARTIAL DENTURE BASE

The denture base functions, to support the artificial teeth and receives the functional forces of occlusion and transfers them to the oral supporting structure. It has following functions.

   i. Provides support to the prosthesis
  ii. Esthetics
 iii. Prevents vertical and horizontal migration of remaining natural teeth
 iv. Eliminates food traps
  v. Stimulate underlying tissue.

The partial denture base may be fabricated in:

- Metal
- Acrylic resin
- Combination of above

Acrylic Resin Base

- Economical and easy to fabricate.
- Relining and rebasing is simple.
- Characterization of resin is possible.
- Esthetics are superior.
- Can be used to support facial tissues like lip and check.
- Easy to repair.
- Latest resin available in variety of materials like monomer free or light cure resins.
- Material of choice for recent extraction cases.

Metal Base

- Accuracy and permanence of form.
- Intimacy of contact with tissue and enhanced retention.
- Stimulates underlying tissue and prevents alveolar atrophy.
- Inherently cleaner, attracts less plaque and calcareous deposits.
- Allows thermal conduction of hot and cold food thereby feels natural.
- Indicated for tooth supported partial dentures and in those distal extension cases where the ridge conditions is stable following many years of extraction.
- Indicated for heavy bite and limited inter-arch spaces.

- Indicated where patient is allergic to acrylic resin.
- Can be made in cobalt-chromium, gold alloy or titanium alloy.

Selection of Prosthetic Teeth for Removable Partial Denture (Table 2.10)

Table 2.10: Selection of anterior teeth			
	Type of Teeth	*Indications*	*Salient features*
Selection of Prosthetic Teeth for Removal Partial Denture			
1.	**Acrylic denture tooth**	i. Most anterior spaces ii. Excellent, when labial contour must be built out with a flange	i. Good esthetics ii. Can be characterized, addition of wear facets, flattening of contacts depth grinding possible iii. Can be directly abutted to the ridge for pleasing appearance iv. Strong in thin sections v. Main disadvantage: low wear resistance
2.	**Porcelain denture tooth**	i. Most anterior spaces with adequate inter-arch spaces ii. Excellent with labial or buccal flange to restore labial contour	i. Excellent esthetics ii. Low strength
3	**Inter change-able facing**	i. Single tooth replacement ii. Deep bite occlusion with reduced inter-ridge space iii. Poor esthetics	i. Strongest of all replacement types ii. Easy to repair
4	**Pressed on/post**	i. Extreme deep bite situation ii. Indications same as that of inter-changeable facing	i. Stronger than acrylic denture teeth ii. Superior esthetics as compared to inter-changeable facing.
Selection of Posterior Teeth			
1	**Resin denture tooth**	i. Opposed to gold surface ii. Opposed to natural teeth iii. Opposed to resin or porcelain teeth	i. Easiest to fit the residual ridge ii. Low wear of opposing dentition iii. Cusp-fossae arrangement possible in anatomic form.
2	**Resin with gold occlusal**	i. Where acrylic teeth are indicated, but will wear of fast due to acrylic poor wear resistance	i. Excellent wear efficiency and resistance to breakage ii. Gold occlusal surfaces are added as modified 3/4th crowns, to acrylic teeth after preparation
3	**Porcelain denture tooth**	i. Opposed to porcelain ii. Opposed to resin teeth	i. Excellent esthetics, and wear resistance ii. Excellent masticatory efficiency iii. Weak in thin sections iv. Difficult to process because of danger of breakage

Contd.

	Type of Teeth		Indications	Salient features
4	**Metal tooth**		i. Restricted posterior space ii. Mesially drifted first molars iii. Edentulous space measuring 3 to 8 mm mesiodistally.	i. Oral hygiene is good. ii. High wear resistance
5	**Pressed on acrylic**		i. Any posterior edentulous space	i. Can be fitted into narrow or short edentulous space. ii. Ample strength iii. Poor esthetics

Methods of Attaching Artificial Teeth to Denture Base (Table 2.11)

	Table 2.11: Methods of attaching artificial teeth to denture base	
1	**Porcelain or acrylic teeth attached with acrylic resin**	Retention of porcelain teeth to acrylic is purely mechanical. Posterior porcelain teeth are retained in their diatoric holes whereas, anterior porcelain teeth are retained by retention pins. Acrylic resin teeth bonds chemically to resin denture base. Attachment of the acrylic resin to the metal base is accomplished by nail head retention, retention loops or diagonal spurs.
2	**Porcelain or Resin tube teeth**	Teeth are adjusted and butted against the ridge to create a ridge lap. The framework is waxed to accommodate custom tooth position. After casting, teeth or facing is cemented with acrylic resin, thereby getting additional reinforcement from metal framework.
3	**Resin teeth processed directly to metal bases**	Modern cross-linked copolymers are used to establish occlusal relationship directly in the mouth on the denture framework.
4	**Metal teeth**	The missing tooth is replaced as part of the partial denture casting.
5	**Chemical bonding**	It consists of direct chemical bonding of acrylic resin to metal framework by following methods. **A. First method:** i. Sand blasting of metal/denture base ↓ ii. Coating of vaporized silica ↓ iii. Application of acrylic resin bonding agent ↓ iv. Acrylic resin **B. Second method:** Tribochemical coating- It consist of: i. Sandblasting of metal with silica particles (Rocatec-Plus) ↓ ii. Silanization of metal framework ↓ iii. 4 META based acrylic resin bonds to metal.

MULTIPLE CHOICE QUESTION

1. **Metal Bases for free end saddle should:**
   A. Not be used
   B. Routinely employed
   C. Restricted to well formed ridges
   D. Stable dental ridges only

2. **Main function of denture base in tooth borne saddle is:**
   A. Tongue massage
   B. Support
   C. Cleanliness
   D. Attachment of artificial teeth

3. **For replacing posterior teeth with RPD, the best choice against natural dentition is:**
   A. Gold occlusal surface
   B. Composite occlusal surface
   C. Acrylic occlusal surface
   D. Chrome-cobalt occlusal surface.

4. **Loss of labial cortex of bone in maxilla is seen commonly in**
   A. Kennedy Class IV
   B. Anterior hyperfunction
   C. Kennedy Class II mod I
   D. Hypertensive patients

5. **The choice of artificial denture teeth for RPD with limited intermaxillary space would be:**
   A. Metal teeth
   B. Tube teeth
   C. Porcelain teeth
   D. Acrylic teeth

6. **For a mandibular distal extension base, border extensions of denture base are best established by:**
   A. Selective pressure technique
   B. Reline technique
   C. Altered cast technique
   D. Kept short of borders as clasp retention is adequate

7. **Reinforced acrylic pontic (RAP) are indicated for:**
   A. Restricted interarch space
   B. Requirement for strength and esthetics
   C. Well healed and contoured residual ridges
   D. All of the above

8 Dentures made with porcelain teeth are easier to rebase
  True/False

9 Porcelain denture tooth should never be used against natural dentition
  True/False

10. The selection of alloy for partial denture framework is based upon all of the following *except*:
   A. Comparative physical properties of alloy
   B. Dimensional accuracy
   C. Availability of the alloy
   D. Patients desire

11. Cobalt chromium framework are preferred over gold framework for RPD primarily due to economic factors. Other advantage of Co-Cr framework is
   A. Stiffness
   B. Hardness
   C. Proportional limit
   D. Yield strength

12. The main disadvantage of using titanium alloys for RPD framework is
   A. Difficulty in casting
   B. Tarnish and corrosion
   C. High cost
   D. Low hardness

13. The undercut requirement for which of the following alloy would be greatest for the same length of clasp?
   A. Titanium alloy
   B. Co-Cr alloy
   C. Ni-Cr alloy
   D. Gold alloy

14. Which of the following is not a technique of attaching artificial teeth to denture base?
   A. Chemical bonding
   B. Cross-linked copolymers
   C. Press on acrylic
   D. Adhesive cementation

15. Which of the following is not an advantage of metal base?
   A. Permanence of form
   B. Thermal insulation
   C. Better mucosal tolerance
   D. Adequate strength and rigidity in thin sections.

NOTES

ANSWERS

1 D Residual ridge reduction is a chronic and continuous process. Metal bases are difficult to reline. Denture bases for free end saddle will require frequent relines. However, those free end ridges which are well formed and have shown positive bone indices (minimal changes over a period of time) can be considered for metal bases.

2 D

3 A

4 B

5 D Dental porcelain teeth cannot be modified gingivally, to any great extent without removing the mechanical diatoric hole necessary for bonding.

6 C

7 D RAP consists of an acrylic resin denture tooth, attached to a centrally located metal reinforcing strut that projects from the removable partial denture framework.

8 True

9 True

10 D

11 A Co-Cr alloy have following mechanical properties
1. Low yield strength
2. Low proportional limit.
3. Greater rigidity → stronger in thin sections, less bulky requires less undercut.
4. Greater hardness → disadvantage as opposing enamel wears faster.
   Gold alloy posses high yield strength, low modulus of elasticity, greater flexibility, high density.
   Gold frameworks are more prone to produce galvanic shocks to abutment teeth restored with dissimilar material.

12 A CP titanium has high affinity for element such as oxygen, nitrogen and hydrogen when in liquid state. Thus it requires an inert atmosphere.
Also, Ti-6Al-4V alloy when used for RPD framework have
1. High yield strength.
2. Modulus of elasticity is higher than gold alloy but lower than Co-Cr and hence they are less rigid.
3. Wrought titanium alloy wires are also flexible.

10 A Titanium alloy have low modulus of elasticity.

14 D

15 B

PRECISION ATTACHMENTS AND STRESS BREAKER

Precision attachment (Synm: parallel attachment, frictional attachment, internal attachment, key and keyway attachment, slotted attachment).

Definition: A direct retainer, used in fixed and removable partial denture construction, consisting of a metal receptacle and a closely fitting part; the former is usually contained within the normal or expanded contours of the crown of the abutment tooth and the latter is attached to a pontic or to the denture framework.

A precision attachment is supposed to be a connecting link between the fixed and the removable type of partial denture because it incorporates features common to both type of construction.

Precision and semiprecision attachments:
1. **Precision attachments** are prefabricated components that are machined to very close tolerance and are made up of precious metal.
2. **Semiprecision attachments** are fabricated in dental laboratory either by casting of wax or plastic pattern. They are also referred to as milled rest, internal rest or precision rest. It consists of dovetail shaped keyway representing female which is built into the proximal portion of wax crown. The stud or male portion is an extension and integral part of Removable Partial Denture.

CLASSIFICATION OF PRECISION ATTACHMENTS
(Figs 2.37A To C)

According to Good kind and Baker (1976) Precision attachments are basically classified as follows:

1. **Intracoronal** are contained within the normal contour of the crown of the tooth. They are of two types:
   i. Resilient
   ii. Non resilient
   • Contained within the normal contour of the crown of the tooth.
2. **Extracoronal are also of two types:**
   i. Resilient
   ii. Non-resilient also referred as **STRESS BREAKERS**
   • Extracoronal attachment may be all or partly contained outside the confines of the crown.

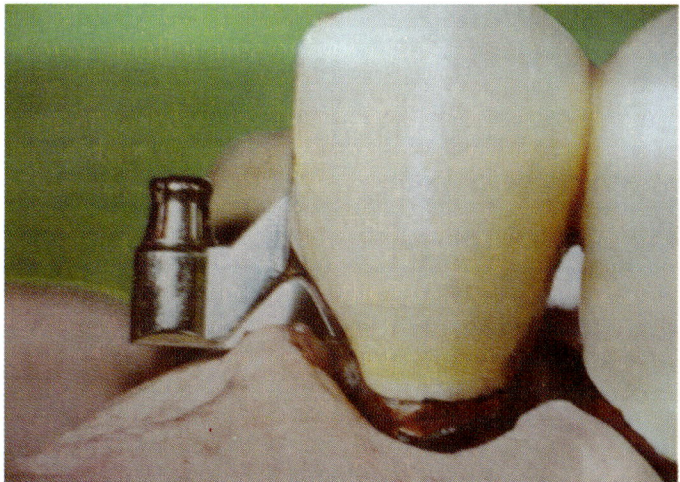

Fig. 2.37A

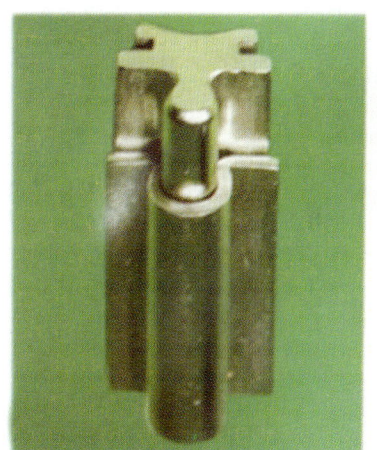
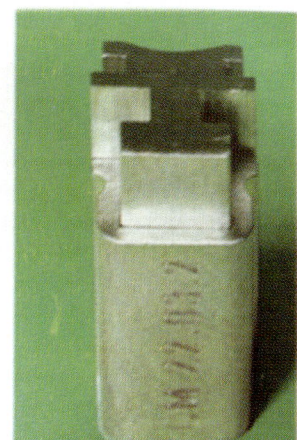

Fig. 2.37B

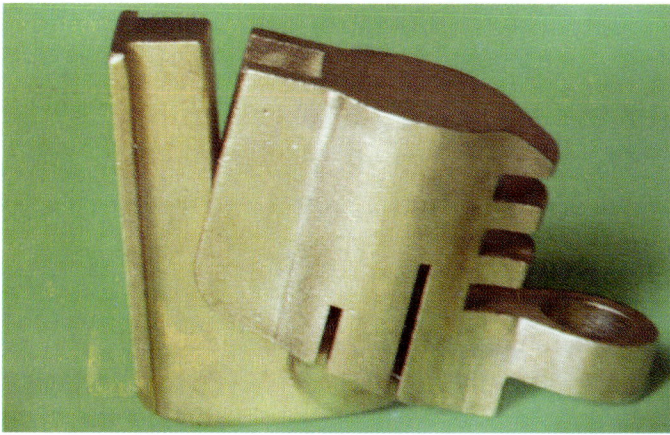

Fig. 2.37C

Figs 2.37A to C: Different types of precision attachments (A) Extracoronal attachment (B) Intracoronal attachments (C) Extracoronal stress breaker attachment

- Extracoronal attachment are used when there is;
  i. Small crown to accommodate the receptacle.
  ii. Pulp chamber is large
- Extracoronal attachment are either in the form of a movable hinge or ball and socket joint, which permits the base to move independent of the retainer.

Purpose of Precision Attachment

The main advantages and rationale behind the use of precision attachment are following:
- High cosmetic excellence
- Elimination of labial/buccal clasp arm
- It directs forces along the long axis of the tooth.
- Intracoronal attachment also provides reciprocation and eliminates whiplash effect.
- It provides an efficient masticatory replacement, through removable and replaceable prosthesis without placing much stress on the abutment teeth.

Indications for the Use of Precision Attachments

- All tooth supported partial dentures
- Free end saddles, stress breakers are used
- Stabilization of teeths, weakened by periodontal disease
- For maximum esthetics

Contraindications for the Use of Precision Attachments

- Teeth with short clinical crowns.
- Teeth that are narrow facio-lingually
- Teeth that have extremely large pulps.
- Lack of patient dexterity or ability to use arm.
- Patient with high caries index

Disadvantages and Limitations of Precision Attachments

- Requires recess preparation for keyway
- Deprives, underlying gingival tissue of customary massage
- The precision attachments greatest wear occurs, during insertion and removal rather than function.
- Friction between the components, could lead to wear and excessive movement of the base and injury/stress to the abutment.
- They are prone to breakage, and difficult to repair

Semi-Precision Attachment

- It consists of narrow slot or keyway with vertical walls, which is built into a casting in an abutment tooth and into which is fitted a male attachment which is a part of RPD framework.
- A lingual clasp arm is must with precision rest, which helps to guide the attachment into place.
- It is simpler to construct, less time consuming and less costly, but lacks high degree of precision.

The Stress Breaker

It is an extracoronal type of precision attachment used with distal extension situations.

It is based upon following concepts:
1. Split major connector (flexibility of the metal framework.)
2. Hinge joint
3. Ball and socket joint

Stress breaker takes off the off-vertical load from the abutment and transfers it to the ridge. They are primarily indicated for:
  i. Weak abutment
  ii. Well formed residual ridge with positive bone factor or index.

Disadvantages of Stress Breaker

1. Excessive alveolar ridge resorption due to lateral forces.
2. Loss of cross arch balance and indirect retention.
3. Bulky, can interfere with teeth arrangement.
4. Food entrapment and difficulty to keep clean.
5. High cost.

MULTIPLE CHOICES QUESTION

1. **The semi-precision attachments differ from precision attachment due to which of the following factor?**
   A. Tapered wall geometry of semi-precision attachment.
   B. Parallel wall geometry of semi-precision
   C. Semi-precision are precisely machined
   D. Semi precision have low degree of error tolerance in manufacturing

2. **When using precision attachment for kennedy Cl III modification I. The path of insertion of prosthesis.**
   A. Parallel to the anterior abutment
   B. Parallel to the posterior abutment
   C. Parallel to all four abutment
   D. None of the above.

3. **Retention provided by intracoronal attachment is due to:**
   A. Resistance to deformation of alloy
   B. Flexibility of alloy
   C. Height of attachment
   D. Friction and binding between components

4. **Extracoronal stress breakers are based upon:**
   A. Broad stress distribution
   B. Broken stress philosophy
   C. Physiologic basing
   D. Functional relines

5. **Which of the following is/are disadvantages associated with the use of attachments?**
   A. Complex design, fabrication and clinical treatment.
   B. Increased cost of treatment
   C. Difficult to maintain and repair
   D. All of the above

6 **Minimum abutment height of 6 mm is necessary for placing intracoronal attachment. Which of the following is best used for assessing available vertical space for attachment?**
   A. Vernier caliper
   B. Wrought wire
   C. Measuring tape
   D. EM gauge

7. **Stress breaker permits movement between:**
   A. Major connector and denture base
   B. Direct retainer and major connector
   C. Direct retainer and denture base
   D. All of the above

8 **All of the following permit stress breaking effect** *except*:
   A. Internal rest
   B. Split major connector
   C. Wrought wire
   D. Hinge joint

9. **The main disadvantage of stress breaker is:**
   A. Enhanced ridge reduction
   B. Uniform stress distribution
   C. Weaker abutment
   D. Preservation of alveolar ridge

10. **Main indication for stress breaker is:**
   A. Weak abutments
   B. Well formed ridges
   C. Positive bone factor
   D. All of the above

11. **The precision attachment should not be used in the distal extension base type of partial denture.**

   True/False

ANSWERS

1 A

2 C

3 D

4 B   Broken stress philosophy consists of mechanical devices or attachments positioned between abutments and extension bases which permits vertical, horizontal and rotational movements of the denture bases relative to abutments.

5 D

6 D

7 C

8 A

9 A

10 D

11 True

The key/keyway mechanism allows no freedom of movement, other than in a vertical plane parallel to the long axis of the tooth.

Biomechanics and Principles of Designing Removable Partial Denture

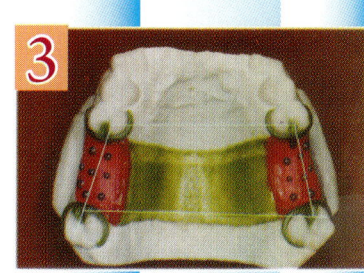

- ❑ Biomechanics and types of lever action
- ❑ Possible movements of partial denture
- ❑ Concepts of designing partial denture
- ❑ Essentials of designing partial denture

BIOMECHANICS

Removable partial dentures are either tooth supported or tooth tissue supported. According to **DeVan,** soft tissue/mucosa is 250 times more displaceable than natural teeth. Successful partial denture prosthesis necessitates mechanical and biological considerations for the purpose of designing.

A class III tooth borne denture behaves much like natural intact arch, by transmitting forces along the long axis. However, distal extension class I or class II and long span class IV removable partial dentures have composite support and are more apt to non-axial loading.

It is this horizontal, oblique, lateral or torquing forces that produces instability and rotational movement of the prosthesis along various planes and axis.

A distal extension prosthesis when subjected to intraoral forces can behave like a lever or an inclined plane. A lever is essentially a rigid bar, supported on above or below somewhere along its length. The support is known as fulcrum.

The lever and inclined plane should be avoided in the design of removable partial denture.

Types of Lever (Fig. 3.1)

1. First class

2. Second class
3. Third class

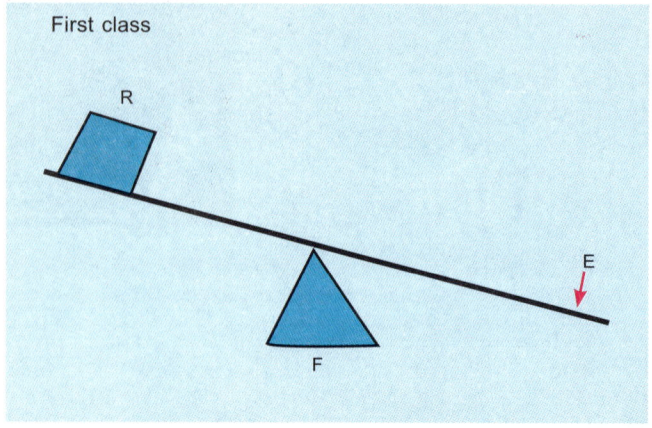

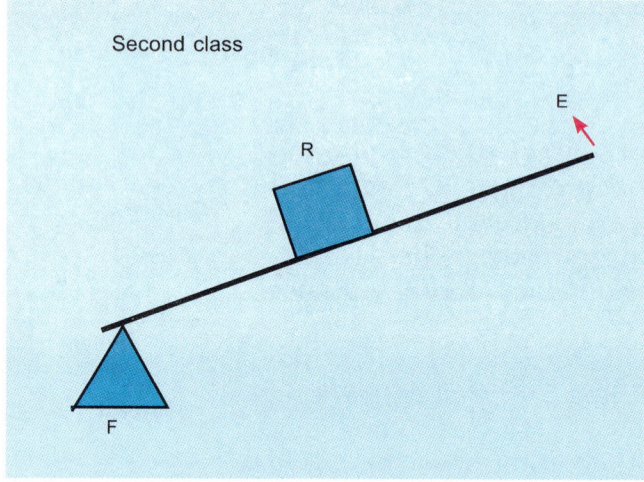

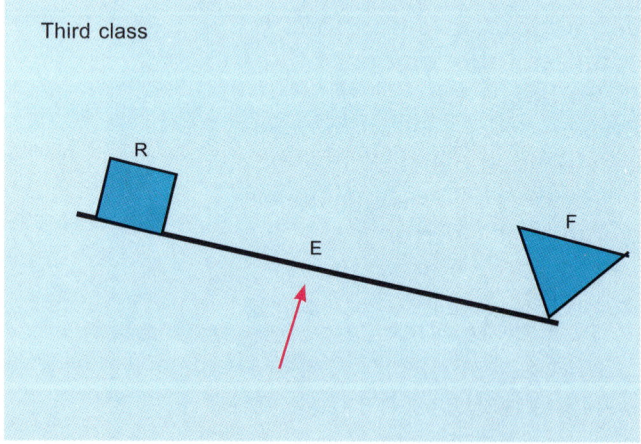

Fig. 3.1: Types of levers possible in partial denture designing depending upon the location of fulcrum, resistance and dislodging force

A distal extension partial denture behaves like a first class lever. As the denture base moves downward under occlusal loads, it rotates about the three fulcrum axis. Simultaneously, off axis loads are transferred to the abutment tooth and soft tissue. Thus, design considerations should incorporate all the necessary components to offset stresses and limit rotational movements of the prosthesis.

Possible Movements of Partial Denture (Fig. 3.2)

Table 3.1	
Sagittal plane	• Rotational movement along the principal fulcrum line passing through the posterior/ main abutments • Movement occurs in sagittal plane either towards or away from the tissue • Resisted by indirect retainers and snow-shoe effect (broad coverage) of the denture base
Frontal plane	• Rotation occurs along the crest of the residual ridge on one side of the arch (longitudinal axis) • Resisted by the rigidity of both major and minor connector.
Horizontal plane	• Rotation occurs around a vertical axis passing through the centre of the arch. Resisted by the stabilising arm and the minor connectors in contact with the vertical tooth structure. Movements in horizontal plane are due to functional and parafunctional forces. They are accentuated by abnormal jaw relationships and disharmonious occlusion. Movement in horizontal plane is present both in tooth supported and tooth tissue supported dentures.

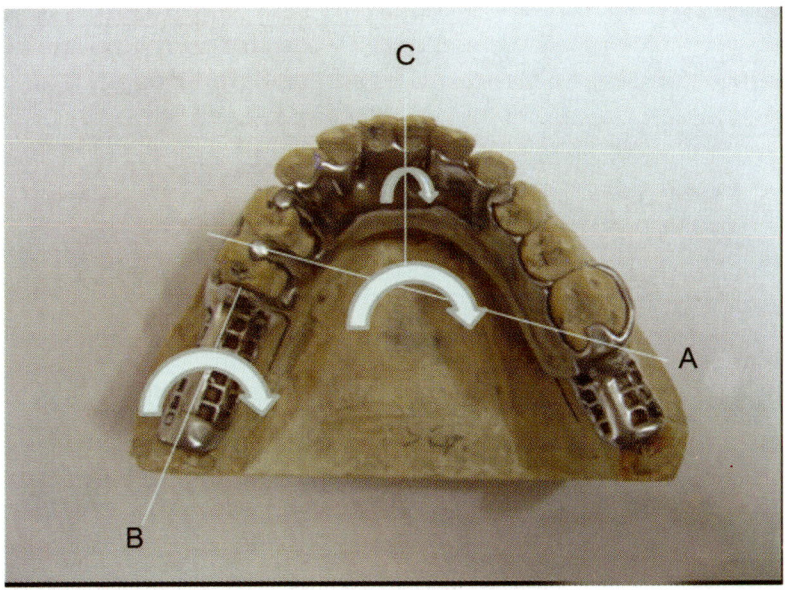

Fig. 3.2: Possible movement of a distal extension partial denture during function. (A) Rotation of the prosthesis along the fulcrum line (B) Rotation of the prosthesis along the crest of the ridge. (C) Rotation of the prosthesis along the vertical axis passing through the centre of the arch

Partial Dentures Design Considerations

A. Concepts of Design (Table 3.2)

Three philosophies exsists behind the designing of cast removable partial denture.

Table 3.2: Concepts of design	
Stress equalization	i. The stresses which are acting upon the distal extension removable partial denture should be directed between the abutment teeth and the edentulous ridge. ii. It advocates non-rigid connection between the denture base and clasp assemblies, e.g. hinge connection. iii. It requires minimal direct retention as the denture bases operate independently.
Physiologic basing	i. It believes in recording the edentulous ridge in its functional form, either by making a functional impression or by functional reline. ii. Functional loading exerts physiological stimulating effect on the tissues of residual ridges. iii. It advocates minimal retention (combination clasp) so as to enhance abutment health. iv. Its disadvantage are occlusal prematurities and less effective indirect retention.
Broad stress distribution	i. Broad coverage by the prosthesis advocates additional rests and clasp assemblies. ii. Total force transmitted over the supporting teeth and mucosa is less. iii. Increased resistance to lateral and horizontal movement. Increased coverage however, complicates oral hygiene.

B. Factors Effecting Stress Generation and Transfer (Table 3.3)

Table 3.3: Allocating stress	
The length of the span	Longer the denture base more leverage will be transmitted to the abutment tooth
Form of residual ridge	Well formed U shaped ridge provides better support and stability
Type of Mucosa	Thin, atrophic and flabby tissues are not preferred
Clasp factor	Flexible clasp transmits more stresses to the residual ridge Balanced clasp having good reciprocation will eliminate the whiplash effect.
Type of abutment surface	Full coverage retainer will offer more frictional resistance than enamel and generate greater stress
Occlusion	Disharmonious occlusion, and the type of prosthesis in the opposing arch will influence the load on removable partial denture. Intact opposing arch will exert greatest forces. Fixed partial denture > Implant supported prosthesis > Removable partial denture will exert forces in the decreasing order on the opposing arch or prosthesis. Complete denture exerts least occlusal forces on the opposing arch

C. Design Considerations (Table 3.4)

The following factors should be taken into considerations whilst designing removable partial denture for better stress allocation and control of prosthesis.

	Table 3.4: Design considerations
i. **Retention**	Clasp retention is the main retention for removable partial denture. However, when other factors of retention like adhesion, cohesion, atmospheric pressure, frictional contact (guide planes), soft tissue undercuts (mylohyoid ridge, tuberosity), neuromuscular forces are utilized the dependency for clasp retention is reduced and also the stress generated.
ii. **Strategic clasp position (Figs 3.3A and B)**	1. **Quadrilateral design**: Four abutments are utilized for clasping. It provides retention, support and stress control. 2. **Tripodal design**: When three clasps; two on tooth supported side and one abutment on distal extension side is used. In tripod design clasps on tooth-borne side should be placed as far away as possible to neutralize the leverage of the distal extension base.
iii. **Clasp design**	Stress release clasps should be preferred for distal extension abutment as mentioned below • Bar clasp • RPI • RPA • Combination clasp • T-bar clasp
iv. **Indirect retention**	An indirect retainer is an element of the removable partial denture that is usually anterior and perpendicular to the fulcrum axis, to counteract the tipping forces which act on the prosthesis when dislodging forces are applied. Indirect retention also help in wider distribution of load and neutralization of stresses. It provides stability and support to the prosthesis.
v. **Occlusion**	• Harmonious occlusion should be developed to minimize off axis loading and trauma to the residual ridge. • Centric relation and centric occlusion should coincide • Teeth should be positioned to favor the weaker ridge. • The size of occlusal table should be reduced.
vi. **Denture base**	• Denture base should extend to cover broader ridge surface for better distribution of stresses. • Denture base should be accurate and stable. • Proper contour and form of polished surface should be established.

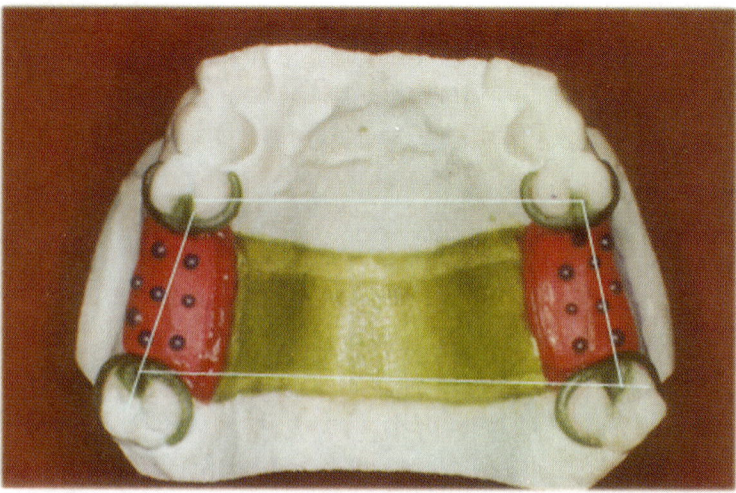

Fig. 3.3A: Quadrilateral clasp arrangement

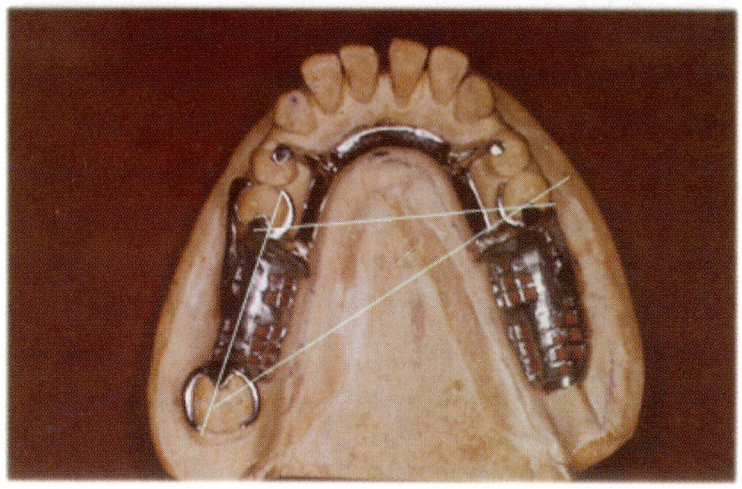

Figs 3.3A and B: Strategic class position

Fig. 3.3B: Tripodal clasp arrangement

ESSENTIALS OF DESIGN (TABLE 3.5)

Table 3.5: Essentials of design	
I. Designing Distal Extension Removable Partial Denture (Kennedy Class I and Class II arches)	
Component	*Reasons for component selection*
i. **Major connector**	Maxillary major connectors are selected for support. When more support from the palate is desired select broader major connector. Mandibular major connector are chosen according to the • Space available • Need for indirect retention.
ii. **Minor connector**	Must be rigid. They are positioned in the embrasure between two teeth and should be inconspicuous to the tongue. Minor connector joining major connector should be rounded to prevent stress concentration and promote patient comfort

Contd.

iii. **Direct Retainer**	Clasp retention should be kept minimal and simplest clasp for a given situation should be chosen. Balanced clasp assemblies where reciprocation, stabilization, retention, encirclement, and support are adequate should be chosen. Wider and strategic clasp positioning, to achieve neutralization of stresses should be achieved **Kennedy Class I** It requires Two clasp one each on two terminal abutment on either side of the arch. Depending upon the location of undercut on terminal abutment the clasp is chosen • Mesiobuccal undercut →RPA, Combination clasp • Mid-buccal→ I-bar, RPI • Disto buccal→ T or modified T bar clasp **Kennedy class II** It requires tripodal clasp configuration: • One clasp on the distal extension side • Two clasp on the opposite side, widely separated as tooth contours and esthetics will permit. Circumferential clasp, on the modification or tooth borne side can be selected
iv. **Indirect retainer**	Indirect retainer is always essential component while designing distal extention base partial dentures. It should be placed anterior and prependicular to the fulcrum axis to control the tipping forces acting on the prothesis when dislodging forces are applied
v. **Rest**	Rest for distal extension should permit ball and socket movement. Rest functions to provide support and directs the forces along the long axis of the abutment. In distal extension mesio-occlusal rest is preferred on the terminal abutment as: • Mesial rest directs the forces anteriorly to other teeth under functional rotation. • It reduces the lever arm and results in more vertical loading of the ridge. • It utilizes greater portion of ridge for support and hence wider stress distribution.

vi. **Occlusion**	• Harmonious occlusion should be achieved.
	• Maximum intercuspation should coincide with centric relation whenever possible.
	• Lateral movements must occur in accordance with remaining natural teeth.
	• Prosthetic teeth should be:
	  i. Fewer and narrower
	  ii. Positioned over the ridge crest
	  iii. Should have sharp cutting edges and sluice ways

vii. **Denture base**	• Should provide:
	  – Broad tissue coverage
	  – Should be accurate and stable
	  – Should be within functional limits
	• Functional relining or selective pressure impression should be utilized for broader coverage and stress distribution
	• Polished surface (cameo) should allow for maximum neuromuscular control

II. Tooth Supported Removable Partial Dentures Design Considerations	
i. **Major and Minor Connector**	Must be rigid and fulfill basic requirements of • Support • Space and location • Indirect retention
ii. **Direct retention**	Quadrilateral clasp arrangement for retention and lateral stability should be considered. Reciprocal arm should be rigid

Contd.

iii.	**Indirect retention**	Usually not required as movement of the prosthesis along the horizontal axis, i.e. fulcrum line is absent
iv.	**Occlusion**	Harmonious occlusion should be achieved. Mostly dictated by the existing natural dentition
v.	**Denture base**	Metal bases are advocated for – Accuracy – Thermal conductivity – As need for relining and rebasing is minimal – Permeance of form

III. Kennedy class IV situation, although tooth-supported, may require following additional considerations.
1. For the reason of esthetics anterior teeth may be arranged anterior to the ridge crest.
2. Acrylic resin denture base is advocated: – To restore labial fullness – To utilize anterior undercut for retention.
3. Indirect retention located posterior to the fulcrum line
4. Quadrilateral Clasp configuration is used and consists of widely separated clasps for retention, stabilization and indirect retention.
5. Functional impression may be indicated if the edentulous area is extensive.

MULTIPLE CHOICE QUESTIONS

NOTES

1. **When designing removable partial dentures for periodontally weakened teeth future design consideration includes which of the following?**
   A. Adequate vertical support maintenance
   B. Ability to add direct retainers
   C. Possibility to reline
   D. All of the above

2. **The first step in designing a removable partial denture is:**
   A. Surveying the primary cast
   B. Outlining the design
   C. Analyzing the oral conditions
   D. None of the above

3. **A properly designed RPD can contribute to oral health. Which of the following conditions can assure long term success with removable partial denture?**
   A. Sound lab procedures
   B. Functional relines
   C. Good oral hygiene protocol
   D. Harmonious occlusion.

4. **A properly designed dentoalveolar and muco-osseous supported distal extension prosthesis will have following number of fulcrum axis:**
   A. One
   B. Two
   C. Three
   D. None

5. **For a distal extension removable partial denture to enhance function which of the following procedure or design features are best desired:**
   A. Altered cast
   B. Dental implant supported prosthesis
   C. Splinting of abutment tooth
   D. All of the above

6. **While outlining the design of a RPD on primary cast which of the following is done last?**
   A. Rest and minor connector
   B. Major connector
   C. Denture bases
   D. Clasp and attachments

7. **Most of removable partial dentures designed world over are done by:**
   A. Specialist doctors
   B. Dental auxiliary
   C. Lab technicians
   D. Dental graduate

8. **Which of the following is the least important component of distal extension RPD?**
   A. Direct retainer
   B. Denture base
   C. Proximal plate
   D. Major connector

9. **During surveying of primary cast, the purpose of fabrication of preparation guide is to shape:**
   A. Rest seats
   B. Major connector
   C. Undercuts
   D. Guiding surfaces

10. **The optimum RPD path of placement:**
    A. Approximates the perpendicular to the plane of occlusion
    B. Is 10 degress Antero-posterior to the path of displacement.
    C. Is when no tooth preparation is required
    D. None of the above

11. **The functions of guiding minor connectors are to:**
    A. Distribute the occlusal load to both sides of the arch
    B. Limit the number of paths of placement and removal
    C. Ensure stability against lateral forces
    D. All of the above

12. **Anterior edentulous spaces are best treated with:**
    A. A fixed partial denture prosthesis
    B. Dental implants
    C. Removable partial denture when soft tissue surgery is indicated
    D. None of the above

NOTES

13. **Which of the following is not a consideration when designing mandibular extension based RPD framework?**
    A. Stress release clasp
    B. Indirect retainer
    C. Support
    D. Mesial occlusal rest

14. **Support from which of the following ridge types would be greater?**
    A. Flat ridge
    B. Sharp spiny ridge
    C. Flabby ridge
    D. Undercut ridge

15. **The contact of proximal plate, over the proximal guide plane in a mandibular distal extension base should be:**
    A. Along the entire length of proximal surface
    B. Upto the junction of middle and gingival third
    C. 1–2 mm on the gingival aspect of guide plane
    D. Middle of middle third

16. **Splint bar RPD frameworks are used for replacing missing anteriors. Which of the following is true for the splint bar denture?**
    A. Made up of 10–13 gauge Co-Cr alloy
    B. Splints remaining anterior teeth
    C. Provides retention, support and stabilization to prosthesis
    D. All of the above

17. **What is a component partial denture ?**

ANSWERS

1 D For periodontally weakened arches following design considerations are suggested.
   a. Multiple rest seats: Provide vertical support and stress distribution.
   b. Use of .0032 nickel chromium wire for use as a retentive arm. It helps in reducing torque.

2 C The first should be to analyze the total oral environment.

3 C

4 D Fulcrum axis line exists only with a poorly fitting RPD.

5 B

6 D

7 C A 1984 survey of removable prosthodontic laboratory in America showed that 78% of removable partial denture are designed by dental technician at the dentist request.

8 A Direct retainer lose their retentive quality within 6 months of usage of RPD due to permanent deformation.
   However, retention from guide planes and proper extension of denture base continues over a longer period.

9 D After tripoding the cast an acrylic resin preparation guide is made to be used in mouth to shape the guiding surfaces and tooth contours and to eliminate undesirable undercuts on the abutment teeth.

10 A

11 D

12 B

13 C Support for distal extension base is accomplished by functional impression techniques more than by the partial denture design

14 A

15 B

16 D Splint bar consists of a anterior rigid bar soldered to adjacent anterior abutments on either side of edentulous region. It provides stability to the removable prosthesis.

17 It is a RPD in which the tooth and tissue portion are fabricated separately and the two are joined with high impact acrylic resin to become a single, rigid functioning unit.

Surveying

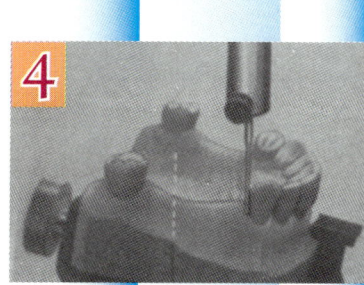

- ❑ Types of surveyor
- ❑ Ney versus Jelenko surveyor
- ❑ Micro analyzer
- ❑ Stress-o-graph
- ❑ Gimble stage table
- ❑ The surveying procedure and the path of insertion

A dental surveyor is essentially a parallelometer used to analyze, the planning cast while designing of the prosthesis. It is used, to determine the relative parallelism of two or more surfaces of the teeth or other parts of the cast of a dental arch.

Dr. A.J. Fortunati was the first person to employ a mechanical device for determining relative parallelism of tooth surfaces by employing a bridge parallelometer. **In 1923, the first commercial dental surveyor was designed by J.M. Ney company of Bloomfield.**

TYPES OF SURVEYOR (Fig. 4.1)

The most commonly used surveyor are Ney and Jelenko. The essential components of each consists of:

i. **Platform** which is parallel to the bench top and give rise to the vertical arm perpendicularly.

ii. **Horizontal arm:** It gives rise to a movable vertical part from which surveying tools are suspended.

iii. **Table** to which cast is attached. The table consists of a ball and socket joint that permits the cast to be oriented in various horizontal planes.

iv. Paralleling tool or guideline marker.

v. Mandrel for holding special tools.
vi. Undercut gauges and tapered tools.
vii. Wax trimmer.

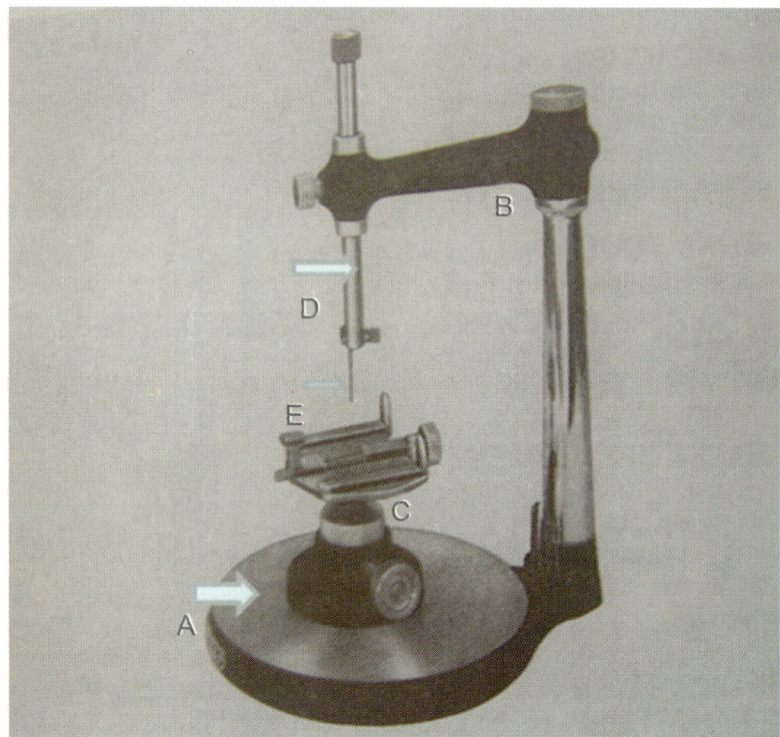

Fig. 4.1: Parts of dental surveyor (A) Platform (B) Horizontal arm (C) Surveyor table (D) Surveying arm (E) Analyzing rod

NEY VERSUS JELENKO SURVEYOR

The basic difference between the Jelenko and Ney Surveyor is that, in Jelenko the horizontal arm can swivel thereby the arm is free to move in horizontal plane rather than depending on the horizontal movement of cast for surveying. Also, in Jelenko the vertical or the surveying arm is spring mounted and in Ney it is friction retained and can be easily used for holding hand piece to cut recesses in cast restorations.

MICROANALYZER

It is a sophisticated surveying instrument that is capable of measuring the amount of undercut electronically in millimeters.

STRESS-O-GRAPH

It is a type of surveyor with two vertical tool holder.

GIMBLE STAGE TABLE

It is used with Williams surveyor. It is that table which is adjustable to any desired anterior, posterior or lateral tilt. The degree of inclination can be recorded for repositioning of cast at any time. The center of rotation of the table is always constant. William's surveyor rod is spring supported. The surveyor is best suited for placement of internal attachments rather than as cast analyzer.

Rationale for Surveying

The surveyor makes it possible to design a removable partial denture, so that resilient and non-resilient section go into place in the mouth as a single unit, free from interferences from either tooth or soft tissue convexities and is capable of resisting dislodging forces in function.

Primary Purpose of Surveying

  i. Assist placement of prosthesis-determines path of insertion and removal.
 ii. Enhances esthetic by selection of right path of insertion and removal.
iii. Resist dislodging forces.
 iv. Eliminates food traps.

Secondary Purpose of Surveying

   i. Surveying the diagnostic cast for effective diagnosis and treatment planning.
  ii. Contouring of wax patterns for locating guide pianes.
 iii. Surveying ceramic veneer crowns.
  iv. Placement of intracoronal precision attachments.
   v. Placement of internal rest/semiprecision attachments.
  vi. Machining of cast restorations.
 vii. Surveying the master cast for path of placement, location of retentive area and location of remaining interferences.
viii. To trim blockout material parallel to the path of placement before duplication.

THE SURVEYING PROCEDURE AND THE PATH OF INSERTION

The surveying procedure focuses attention on the following four factors which are the key stone of partial denture design. The interplay of these four factors influences the path of insertion for the prosthesis.

The factors are:

1. Guide planes
2. Retentive undercuts
3. Interferences
4. Esthetics.

1. Guide Planes (Fig. 4.2)

1. Guiding planes are the axial surfaces of teeth which are contacted by the rigid elements of the prosthesis as it is seated and removed from the mouth.
2. Guide planes ensure predictable clasp assembly function.
3. Provides bracing, stabilization and retention.

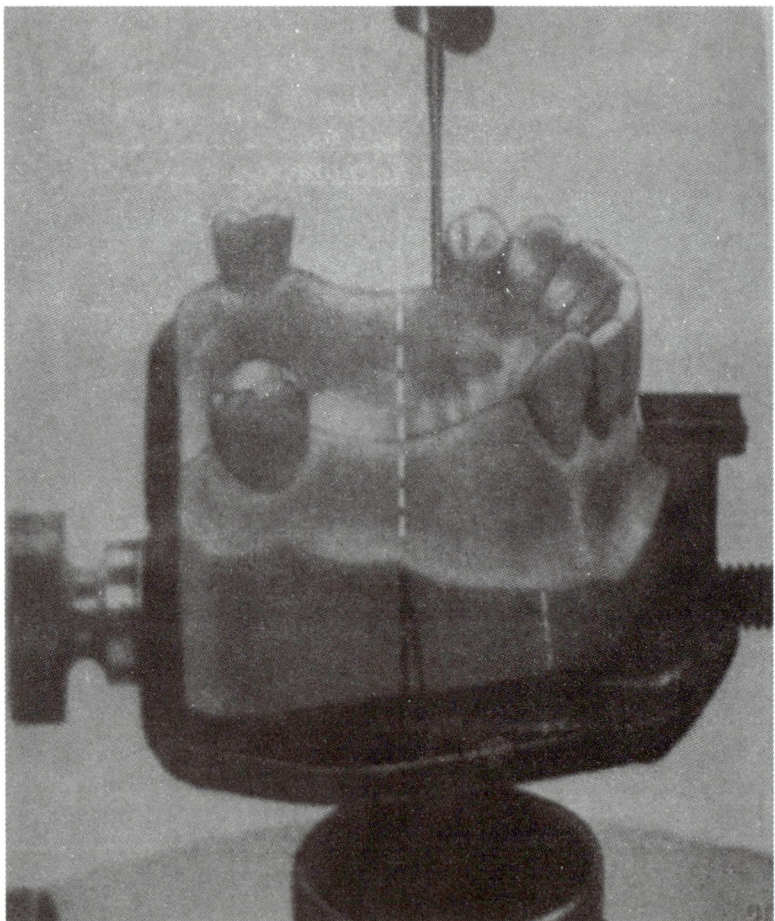

Fig. 4.2: Guide planes

4. The surveyor helps in identifying proximal and other axial surfaces of the abutment teeth, which can be prepared parallel to each other by altering or by addition of restoration for unimpeded passage of the prosthesis along the established path of insertion.

2. Retentive Area (Figs 4.3A and B)

Retentive area must exist for a given path of placement. Buccal and lingual surface of principal abutment teeth are surveyed and undercut area identified below the height of contour.

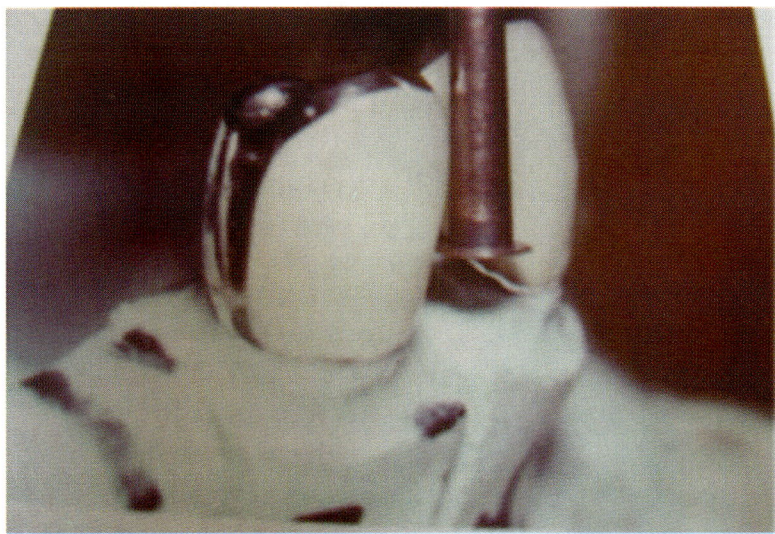

Fig. 4.3A

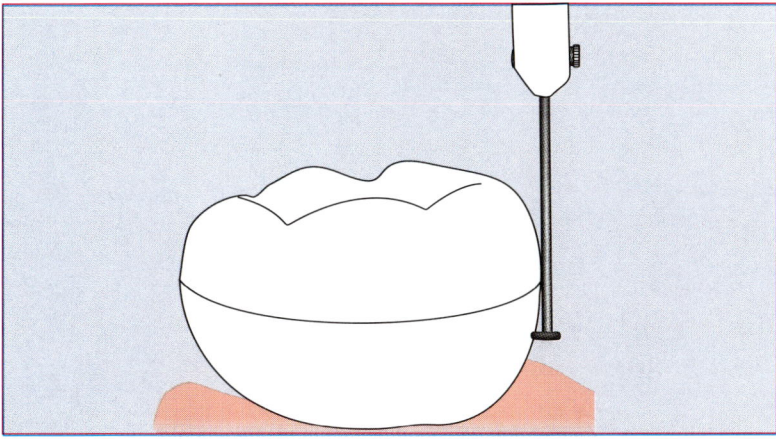

Fig. 4.3B

Figs 4.3A and B: Retentive area

The retentive undercut may be visualized as having three dimensions
  a. Mesio-distal
  b. Bucco-lingual
  c. Occluso-gingival
Bucco-lingual dimension gives the amount of depth of undercut (Horizontal). It is important, because as the clasp terminal enters or leaves the infrabulge area it should flex an amount equal to the depth of undercut. The accurate measurement of the undercut on an abutment tooth is an exacting procedure. The shank of the undercut gauge should contact the height of contour of the tooth at the same time that the undercut gauge contacts the surface of the tooth in the undercut.

Amount of Undercut required for:

- Cobalt-chromium : 0.010″ for bicuspid
  clasp   0.015″ for molars
- 18 gauge gold   : 0.020″ inch
  wire clasp

3. Interferences

Certain areas of patient mouth may present interferences to easy insertion and removal of prosthesis. They are both hard tissue and soft tissue obstacles.

Hard Tissue Interferences

- Migrated, tipped and rotated teeth
- Splayed molars
- Teeth with high survey line, e.g. disto buccal line angles of the maxillary bicuspids, mesiobuccal line angles of the maxillary molars and mesiolingual line angles of mandibular molars.

Soft Tissue Interferences

- Mylohyoid ridge prominence.
- Prominent tuberosity.
- Mental region area.
- Labial ridge undercuts.
  Interferences can be identified by surveying the cast and can be treated by either.
  a. Elimination (extraction).
  b. Alteration (disking, surgery, restorations).

c. Avoidance (modification of design).

d. Exploitation (using an exsisting undercut for prosthesis retention).

4. Esthetics

Path of placement also influences esthetic of the denture by influencing location of clasp and arrangement of teeth. Gingivally approaching clasp have better esthetics then occlusally approaching.

Path of Placement

The path of insertion may be defined as the direction in which the restoration is placed and removed from the basal seat. Path of insertion is different from path of displacement of prosthesis.

Path of displacement of prosthesis is always perpendicular to the occlusal plane of the patient. However, path of insertion may be arcuate or any other and is governed by guide planes and clasp assembly.

Path of insertion is influenced by the type of prosthesis

Tooth bound prosthesis: Single path of insertion and removal.

Distal extension type: Two or more path of insertion one perpendicular to plane of occlusion and other arcuate path which it follows as the clasp rotates on the abutment teeth.

Cast Tilting for Surveying (Figs 4.4A and B)

i. The tilt of the cast refers to the position of the cast on the surveyor table relative to the horizontal plane, at the time prosthesis is designed.

ii. Tilting the cast on surveyor table changes the long axis of each tooth relative to the horizontal plane. Also survey line, location of retentive and non-undercut areas can be modified.

iii. The path of insertion and path of displacement of prosthesis may not be the same. For the prosthesis to be retentive, the resistance of a clasp to dislodgement must be effective at right angles to the occlusal plane, regardless of the path of insertion.

iv. Retentive undercut must exist with the cast in horizontal position.

v. Cast tilting is of advantage when extreme labial under-cut exist anteriorly in Kennedy Class IV situation. By utilizing an anterior path of insertion labial undercuts and guide plane can be used to design snugly fitting prosthesis.

vi. No, more than 15 degrees of anterior-posterior tilting is permissible while surveying.

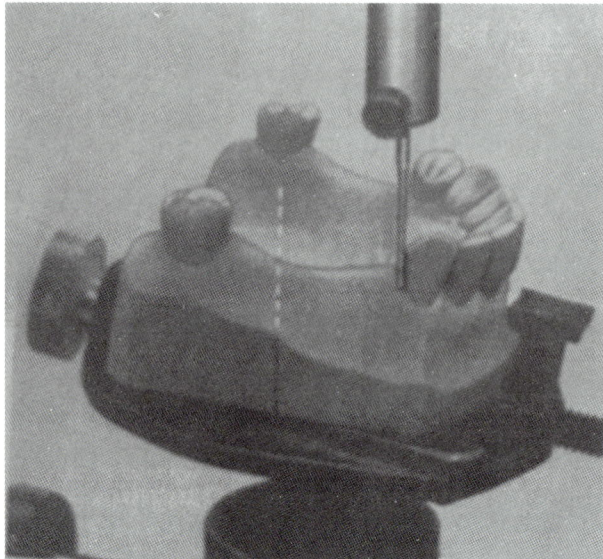

Fig. 4.4A: Anterior tilt

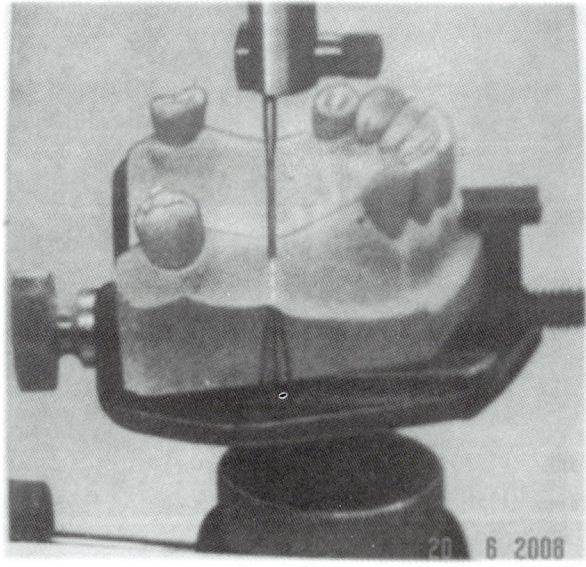

Fig. 4.4B: Posterior tilt

Figs 4.4A and B: Cast tilting for surveying

Tripoding

It is a procedure of indexing the partial denture cast, which allows the cast to be returned to the same horizontal plane in which it is surveyed without loss of orientation during the process of designing of removable partial denture.

Tissue Surface Tripoding

Three distinct widely separated locations are marked with lead in the surveyor spindle on the tissue surface of the cast. These marks exist at same horizontal position, thus, the plane of surveying gets recorded or indexed.

Art Portion Tripoding

It is done with the analyzing rod held against the art portion of the cast. Three lines are drawn with lead marker, one on the posterior aspect and one each on the lateral aspect.

Tripoding preserves the tilt of the cast and fixes the plane of cast decided for designing. It allows the casts to be removed and returned to its original position whenever desired.

Use of Surveyor (Table 4.1)

Table 4.1: Purposes of surveyor	
Primary purpose	Analyze the primary cast for • Claspability • Interferences • Esthetics • Guide planes
Secondary purpose	• Survey lines • Undercut depth • Tripodization • Contour wax pattern • Contour restorations
Auxillary uses	• Shaped blockout • Precision, semiprecision attachments placement • Check parallelism in fixed partial denture • Determine need for alveoloplasty in complete denture.

MULTIPLE CHOICE QUESTION

1. **Dental surveyor acts as/to:**
   A. Parallelometer
   B. Correlates resilient and non-resilient components
   C. Determine most advantageous cast position
   D. All of the above

2. **Which of the following was the first surveyor designed commercially?**
   A. Ney
   B. Jelenko
   C. Wills
   D. Micro analyzer

3. **Primary surveying is done to:**
   A. Locate undercuts
   B. Measure undercuts
   C. Outline design of RPD
   D. None of the above

4. **The first commercial surveyor was designed by**
   A. Weinsten and Roth
   B. Applegate
   C. A.J. Fortunati
   D. Kennedy

5. **Which of the following situations will have more than one path of insertion?**
   A. Kennedy class II
   B. Kennedy class I
   C. Kennedy class II mod I
   D. All of the above

6. **Which of the following is not a factor of path of insertion?**
   A. Guiding planes
   B. Retentive undercuts
   C. Position of survey line
   D. Esthetics

7. **Dental cast for surveying should not be tilted more than:**
   A. 5°
   B. 10°
   C. 15°
   D. 20°

8. **Tripoding of dental Cast:**
   A. Preserves the tilt/orientation
   B. Not necessary for class III arches

C. Determines path of insertion

D. Locates retentive undercuts

9. **Surying is least important in the fabrication of:**
   A. Removable partial dentures
   B. Fixed partial dentures
   C. Complete removable dentures
   D. Implant dentures
   E. None of the above

10. **Which component of dental surveyor determines parallelism?**
    A. Analyzing rod
    B. Carbon marker
    C. Wax trimmer
    D. Vertical arm

11. **First area in mouth preparation which can prevent incomplete seating of cast partial denture:**
    A. Proximal guide plane
    B. Retentive undercut
    C. Sharp marginal ridge
    D. All of the above

12. **Function's of guide plane are all except**
    A. Horizontal stabilization
    B. Increase retention
    C. Stress release
    D. Support

13. **Which of the following is not true for proximal guide plane?**
    A. Flat occluso gingivally
    B. Follow facio-lingual contour
    C. Parallel to path of insertion
    D. 6 mm occlusogingivally

14. **The best method for achieving retentive undercut in cases where none exsists at 0° tilt would be:**
    A. Dimpling
    B. Tilting the cast
    C. Cast crowns
    D. Modification of survey lines

15. **Which of the following regarding occlusal rest seat in posterior teeth is true?**
    A. 3-4 mm mesial to distal
    B. Facio-lingually half the distance between cusp tips

C. Spoon shaped floor
D. Triangular outline form
E. Floor should be perpendicular to the long axis
F. All of the above

16. **Long box rests are indicated in:**
    A. Distal extension RPD's
    B. Rotational path RPD's
    C. Stress breaker concept
    D. None of the above

17. **For Rotational path RPD's which of the following is true?**
    A. Long box rests
    B. Rigid direct retainers
    C. Dual path of insertion
    D. Esthetics and less metal display
    E. All of the above

18. **Esthetics of a removable partial denture is primarily determined by**
    A. Characterized denture bases
    B. Dentogenic concept of teeth selection
    C. Elimination of retentive arm
    D. Path of placement

19. **Final path of placement of RPD prosthesis is:**
    A. Anterio-Posterior tilt of the cast
    B. Lateral tilt of cast
    C. Combination of A-P and lateral tilt
    D. zero degree tilt

20. **The purpose of surveying the master cast during fabrication of RPD is all of the following *except*:**
    A. Delineate height of contour
    B. Measure retentive undercut
    C. Block out unwanted undercuts
    D. Establish the path of insertion

21. **Parallel block out is done on which of the following areas of master cast?**
    A. Guiding planes
    B. Beneath minor connectors
    C. Major connector area
    D. All of the above

ANSWERS

1 D
2 A
3 D
4 A
5 B
6 C
7 B
8 A
9 E
10 A
11 C
12 D
13 D
14 C
15 F
16 B
17 E
18 D
19 C
20 D
21 D All areas that will be contacted by rigid parts of denture framework must be made free of undercuts by parallel block out.

Examination, Diagnosis, Treatment Planning, Mouth and Abutment Preparation for Removable Partial Denture

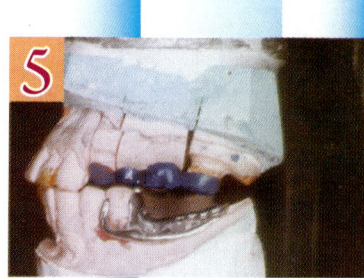

- ❑ Optimum treatment
- ❑ Occlusal considerations
- ❑ Tooth alteration procedures

Removable Partial denture treatment service should fulfil following objectives:

i. Complete elimination of disease.
ii. Preservation, restoration and maintenance of the health of remaining teeth and oral tissue. To distribute load equally between the teeth and associated alveolar ridge.
iii. Satisfactory replacement of missing natural teeth and tissue.
iv. Restoration of function, esthetic and patient comfort to optimum.

The treatment plan for a given case should be established beforehand the definitive treatment. Patients examination, diagnosis and treatment plan should follow a definitive sequential order.

OPTIMUM TREATMENT

Diagnostic clinical examination
↓
Treatment plan
↓
Definitive treatment

Diagnostic, Clinical Examination and Treatment Planning

Following is the list of clinical findings and its significance on the treatment planning of partially edentulous arches (Table 5.1).

Table 5.1	
Clinical finding	*Significance*
1. **Systemic condition**	
a. Controlled	• Good prognosis • Good tissue tolerance
b. Uncontrolled	• Poor tissue tolerance • Added stress on abutment teeth • Poor prognosis of prosthesis
2. **Oral hygiene**	• Oral health care education, motivation and periodic observation • Uncontrolled plaque and calculus deposits contradicts removable partial denture service.
3. **Anatomic interferences like Tori, prominent mylohyoid ridge, others**	• Palatal tori can be bypassed in design of major connector. • Mandibular tori should be surgically removed. • Prominent mylohyoid ridge should be surgically corrected. • Soft permanent lined denture bases can be considered.
4. **Parafunctional habits**	• Transmits horizontal destructive forces on teeth and residual ridge. • Instability of removable partial denture is a major concern.
5. **Periodontal tissue**	• Healthy gingiva is coral pink, translucent, dull and stippled in appearance. • Periodontal therapy for elimination of pockets and correction of recession, should be undertaken prior to removable partial denture fabrication.

6. **Interproximal food impaction**	• There are two types of food impaction
	  i. **Vertical:** Forceful wedging of food against gingival tissue through occlusal pressure.
	  ii. **Horizontal:** Forcing of food between the teeth by the tongue, lip and cheek pressure.

7. **Examination of teeth**	
a. Pulp vitality	• Check vitality by thermal and electronic means of abutment tooth and teeth with deep restorations.
b. Dental caries	• Carious teeths must be restored before starting definitive treatment

c. Mobility
  i. < 1 mm upto 1 mm
  ii. > 1 mm
 	
  iii. Vertical movement
	• Excellent abutment support
	• Surgical therapy and re-evaluation. If mobility decreases can be used as abutment.
	• Extraction

d. Extruded teeth
  i. Slight
  ii. Medium
  iii. Extreme
	• Enameloplasty
	• Onlay restoration is indicated
	• Endodontic therapy/extraction

Contd.

Clinical finding	Significance

e. Shape and length of crown
  i. Insufficient crown height
  ii. Lacks undercut
	• Surgical crown lengthening
	• Full coverage retainer/dimpling/Class V restoration.

f. Abnormal inclinations	• Reshaping and recontouring for modifying height and contour.
g. Length of time since missing	• Check for abnormal chewing patterns, temporomandibular joint problems, jaw deviations and poor attitude of patients.
8. **Radiographic examination**	

a. Lamina dura
  i. absence
  ii. uneven
  iii. thinning
  iv. uninterrupted
	• Indicates periodontitis/bone loss
	• Tooth migration/tilting
	• Periodontal disease
	• Good prognosis

b. Impacted, residual roots/teeth	• Surgical extraction • Impacted molars should be informed about to the patient and retained in younger patients for development of tuberosity ridge form for future support.

c. **Bone Index area**
  Index areas are those areas of alveolar support that discloses the reaction of bone to additional stress.
  i. Positive bone factor
  ii. Negative bone factor
	i. Positive bone factor
	  • Dense cortical bone, dense lamina dura, fine trabeculae pattern.
	ii. Negative bone factor
	  • Bone will respond unfavourably to stress
	  • Poor support.
	  • Resorb faster under occlusal loads.

d. Shape and length of roots
  i. Small, conical roots
  ii. Multi rooted, broad roots
	May need splinting
	Good prognosis, can be used favourably for removable partial denture abutment.

9 **Residual ridge area**	

a. Size and form
  i. Full rounded
  ii. Narrow, flat
  iii. Tuberosity undercut and low
	• Good support
	• Poor support
	• Surgical correction is required

b. Hyperplastic tissue	• Tissue conditioning, finger massage therapy or surgical correction.
c. Interarch space is inadequate	• Surgery required to obtain space for denture base and artificial teeth.

Contd.

	Clinical finding	Significance
10.	**Esthetics**	
	a. Lip	• Evaluate lip support • Lip contour determines labial flange thickness
	b. Shade selection	• Should be done at the time of examination
	c. Diastema between anterior teeth	• It influences upon the design of major connector (step back/cut back design).
11.	**Occlusion**	• Gross occlusal equilibration, should be done before fabrication of Removable partial denture • Plane of occlusion should be established. • Final equilibration is done for obtaining centric occlusion after the prosthesis is ready.
12.	**Interocclusal space**	• Should be sufficient. Areas of abutment teeth that are to receive rests must be evaluated for space.
13.	**TMJ dysfunction**	• Clicking, pain, and joint tenderness, should be ruled out.
14.	**Selection of abutment**	
	a. Molars and cuspids	• Best abutments for stability and strength.
	b. Bicuspids	• Better claspability then cuspids.
	c. Incisors	• Poor abutments
	d. Pier abutments	• Poor abutments (isolated abutment)
	e. Tipped teeth	• Long occlusal rest or crowns required.
15.	**Patient attitude towards a new removable partial denture**	
	a. Philosophic	• Good prognosis
	b. Emotional	• Nervous and temperamental; feels he or she can never wear denture
	c. Exacting	• Perfectionist, difficult patient to satisfy
	d. Indifferent	• Most difficult post insertion patient.

Purpose of Mounted Diagnostic Cast

Patients maxillary diagnostic cast should be mounted in relation to the axis-orbital plane, to permit better interpretation of the plane of occlusion in relation to the horizontal plane. Mandibular cast is then related to the maxillary cast through centric interocclusal record.

Purpose

i. Diagnostic cast provides an opportunity to evaluate the relationship of remaining oral structure.

ii. Identification and location of deflective occlusal contacts.

iii. Visualization of disrupted occlusal plane and tooth migration requiring correction before fabrication of prosthesis.

iv. Assessment of degree of alteration required for recontouring, repositioning or elimination of extruded teeth.

v. Duplicate diagnostic casts are used for marking. Removable Partial denture design and areas needing modifications and tooth preparation.

Mouth Preparations for Removable Partial Dentures

Mouth preparations are those procedures that changes or modifies existing oral structure or conditions to

- Facilitate the placement and removal of the prosthesis.
- Facilitate its physiologic functioning.
- Enhance prosthesis long-term success.

Objectives of Mouth Preparation

i. Establish optimum health of the supporting and contiguous tissues.

ii. Eliminate interferences/obstruction in the path of placement and removal.

iii. To establish an acceptable occlusal scheme and occlusal plane.

iv. To alter, natural tooth form to accommodate the requirements of form and function of the prosthesis.

Mouth preparation are based upon patients clinical examination, radiographic evaluation and surveying of the diagnostic cast. Mouth preparations, are usually carried out after the design of the prosthesis is finalized and all soft tissues and hard tissues abnormalities are corrected.

Mouth preparations for receiving removable partial dentures prosthesis and broadly of two types:

A. Occlusal Considerations

   i. Correction and establishment of occlusal plane.
  ii. Establishing occlusal scheme.

B. Alterations/Modification of Natural Tooth Contours

    i. Establishing guide planes
   ii. Modification of survey lines
  iii. Elimination of interferences
   iv. Preparation of rest seats
    v. Creating undercuts
   vi. Surveyed crowns and crown ledges.

A. OCCLUSAL CONSIDERATIONS

Occlusal plane should be evaluated on mounted diagnostic cast. If the maxillary arch is completely edentulous and the lower arch need a partial removable prosthesis, occlusal templates curved 20 (Trubyte, Dentsply). can be used to analyze irregular occlusal curve on diagnostic cast. Location and magnitude of discrepancies in occlusal curve are noted and recorded.

Occlusal plane discrepancies could be due to either supraerupted teeth or infraerupted teeth.

Supraerupted Teeth (Table 5.2)

Problems due to supraerupted teeth are:
- Insufficient space for framework and artificial teeth placement.
- Occlusal trauma and interferences

Table 5.2: Classification and treatment of supra erupted posterior teeth		
Classification	*Degree of extrusion*	*Treatment required*
Class I	Slight	None
Class II	Moderate	Enameloplasty
Class III	Moderately severe	Complete cast restorations or Endodontic therapy and cast restoration.
Class IV	Severe	1. Repositioning by orthodontics
		2. Endodontic therapy followed by its usage as over denture abutment for support
		3. Extraction
Class V	Complete extrusion contacting opposing ridge mucosa	Extraction/Ro rehabilitative treatment possible (None)

- Extruded teeth in the anterior region causing esthetic problems.

Infraerupted Teeth

They can be corrected by:
- Orthodontic extrusion
- Cast restoration
- Occlusal onlay or overlay restorations.

ii. Occlusal Scheme

1. When there are insufficient tooth contacts present to provide a stable inter-cuspal position, occlusion should be adjusted to achieve harmony between the retruded contact position and the intercuspal position in the finished removable partial denture.
2. If the patient's exsisting dentition is free of pathosis and sufficient natural teeth remains, then patients existing occlusion should be chosen for establishing the occlusal scheme of removable partial denture.

B. TOOTH ALTERATION PROCEDURES

i. Guide Planes Preparation (Figs 5.1A and B)

Definition	Naturally occurring/prepared parallel areas on vertical tooth surfaces that are contacted by certain rigid parts of the removable partial denture framework during the placement and removal of the prosthesis.
Purpose	To establish a single, predictable path of placement and removal.
Configuration	
Length	Longer occlusogingivally for tooth supported than for distal extension prosthesis.
Proximal	They extend from marginal ridge cervically. **Tooth supported:** 1/2 to 2/3rd occlusogingivally. **Tooth tissue supported:** 1/3rd to 2/3rd occluso gingivally
Width	When viewed occlusally the proximal guide planes extends buccolingually and follow natural tooth contours, slightly curved. Canines/premolars: 3 to 4 mm wide Molars: 4 to 5 mm wide

Guide planes are also prepared on other axial surfaces with smooth diamond stone (cylindrical/tapered) by keeping the long axis parallel with the path of placement.

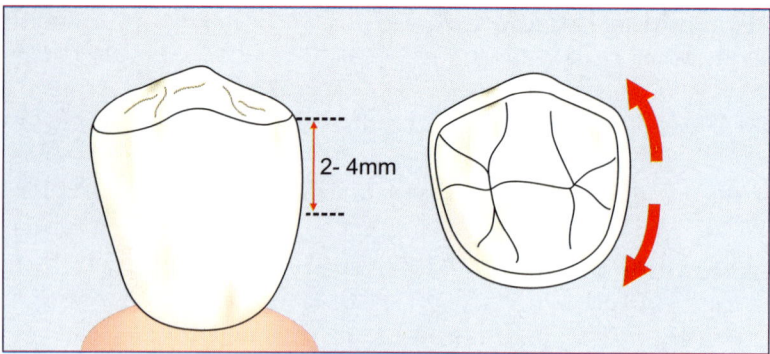

Fig. 5.1A: Guide plane adjacent to tooth supported saddle should extend 2–4 mm occlusogingivally

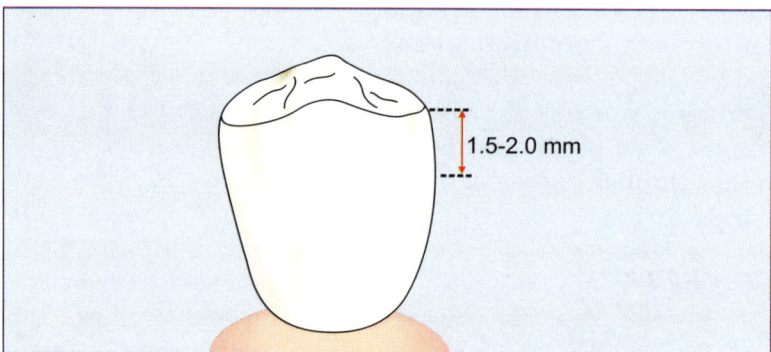

Figs 5.1A and B: Guide plane preparation

Fig. 5.1B: Guide plane adjacent to distal extension saddle should be 2 mm occlusogingivally

ii. Modification of Survey Line/Height of Contour

Survey line can be modified by:
a. Changing the tilt of cast
b. Selective grinding/enameloplasty
c. Cast restorations

- Modification of survey line by changing the cast tilt should be done before final diagnostic cast position is selected. Cast tilting modifies survey line on all the teeth.
- Enameloplastly can be used to achieve, favorable survey line on one particular/abutment tooth.
- Survey lines can be lowered but not raised by selective grinding.
- Modification of survey line is desirable for
  – Appropriate clasp placement
  – Proper location of shoulder, reducing the degree of undercut and proper placement of reciprocal arm.

- Modification procedures should only be limited to enamel and not expose dentin.

iii. Elimination of Interferences

Interferences to path of placement and removal are encountered from the teeth, and the associated soft tissues.

Interferences from the teeth are due to divergent axis, malposed, tipped or atypically contoured teeth.

Soft tissue interferences are usually associated with a bony component and are usually in the form of tori, bony undercut, or anatomic landmark like mylohyoid ridge.

Interferences, can be
- Eliminated (extraction-ablation)
- Altered (disking, surgery, restoration)
- Avoidance (modification of design)
- Exploitation (using an undercut to help retain the prosthesis).

iv. Preparation of Rest Seat

Rest seat/rest areas are specially prepared tooth surfaces designed to accommodate the metal rest of the removable partial denture framework. Rest seat preparation should follow all selective grinding procedures like preparation of guide plane, lowering/modification of survey lines.

Two main type of rest are common:
a. Intracoronal: Rest prepared in a restoration such as a crown or inlay
b. Extracoronal: Rest placed on natural or restored tooth surfaces.

Extracoronal Rest are of various types:
- Occlusal
- Incisal
- Cingulum
- Combinations—e.g. proximal occlusal rest, embrasure occlusal rest, embrasure incisal rest, proximal incisal hook rest.

Rest should be ideally prepared in sound enamel. Sometimes rest seats are also placed in existing restorations.

Gold and gold substitutes are the most acceptable restorative material to support rest. Rest can also be prepared in amalgam and dental porcelain surfaces.

Functions of Rest

- Serves, as vertical stops in the final seating of the prosthesis
- Maintains predictable clasp position.
- Prevents soft tissue impingement.
- Directs occlusal forces along the long axis of the abutment teeth.
- Prevents abutment tooth extrusion.
- Serves as indirect retainer.
- Deflect food away from tooth contacts and embrasure spaces.

v. Creating Undercuts (Fig. 5. 2)

Once the final path of insertion and removal of the prosthesis has been chosen, the shape of abutment tooth may not present acceptable undercuts for clasp retention. A technique known as dimpling or grooving may be employed which consists of preparing a small indentation in the enamel of the tooth surface into which will fit a small boss (rounded tip) of the retentive tip. It is 0.010 to 0.015 inch excavation which is saucer shaped and prepared in the interproximal area where the enamel is thick. Dimpling is mainly indicated for

- Mandibular cuspids where no undercuts exists.
- Patient for cosmetic reason or otherwise do not wish to have full coverage restorations done.
- The area of location of dimple should be parallel to the path of placement.
- It can also be placed on the previously restored tooth surface ideally in gold and gold substitutes.

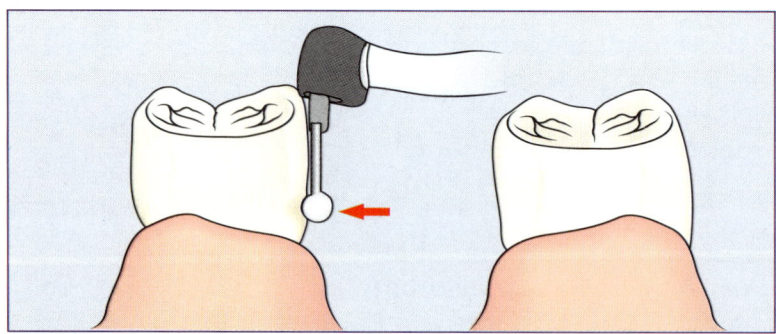

Fig. 5.2: Creating undercut (Dimpling) with round bur in sound enamel

vi. Surveyed Crown and Crown Ledges

Surveyed crowns are cast restorations that are fabricated for teeth serving as abutments for removable partial dentures. The restorations while they are being fabricated, are surveyed for guide planes, survey lines, retentive undercut and rest seat preparation. Conventional crown preparation need to be modified to meet the design requirement of surveyed crowns. The reduction of additional tooth surface is usually required in the following instance:

- To cut/recess for rest seat
- To shorten the clinical crown
- To reduce severe interferences and undercuts
- To develop appropriate guide planes
- To provide adequate space for the artificial teeth, by correction of plane of occlusion.

Crown ledge, is a form of a lingual ledge rest placed in the crown retainer of abutment tooth. It is cut in the wax up stage parallel to the path of placement. It acts like a precision guide plane. It also provides reciprocation and eliminates the need of reciprocal arm.

MULTIPLE CHOICE QUESTIONS

1. **Covert examination refers to:**
   A. Physical examination of the patient
   B. Radiographic examination
   C. Study cast analysis
   D. Observation of patient's behaviour

2. **Contigency design of removable partial denture indicates**
   A. Interim prosthesis
   B. Transitional prosthesis
   C. Definitive prosthesis
   D. None of the above

3. **During examination of a patient for fabrication of mandibular removable partial denture lingual tori are observed. The treatment planning best suited for such a case is:**
   A. Relief over tori
   B. Labial major connector
   C. Termination of lingual bar above the superior end of tori
   D. Swing lock partial denture

4. **Severe bilateral tuberosity undercuts when present during fabrication of maxillary distal extension cast partial dentures are treated by:**
   A. Surgical removal of both undercuts
   B. Use of resilient liners for denture base
   C. Termination of denture base short of tuberosity
   D. Removal of one undercut and utilization of other by rotational path of denture insertion.

5. **With high positioned mandibular lingual frenum the choice of mandibular major connector would be:**
   A. Lingual bar
   B. Labial bar
   C. Linguo plate
   D. Double linguo bar

6. Bone index factors, are good indicator of support ability of alveolar bone adjacent to teeth subjected to high stress levels:

   True/false

7. Mounted diagnostic cast provides crucial information about a situation requiring prosthetic service. Which of the following information is not provided by them?
   A. Occlusal interferences
   B. Plane of occlusion
   C. Inter ridge space
   D. Inter occlusal space
   E. All of the above

8. The first main step, before treatment with partial denture is initiated is the
   A. Correction of occlusal plane
   B. Establishment of guide plane
   C. Rest seat preparation
   D. Removal of interferences by enameloplasty

9. RPD are subjected to various stresses and rotational movements. Most damaging forces on a removable partial denture is exerted by:
   A. Functional closure while chewing
   B. Parafunctional forces
   C. Strain from clasp placement and removal
   D. All of the above

10. Most common cause of failure of removable partial denture is:
    A. Inadequate support for denture bases
    B. Failure to develop a harmonious occlusion
    C. Faulty surveying of cast
    D. Improper diagnosis and treatment planning.

11. Single most critical factor for the success of RPD service is:
    A. Adequate plaque control
    B. Proper diagnosis and treatment planning
    C. Framework distortion
    D. Inadequate denture base extension

NOTES

12. **RPD design should be established and recorded on the mounted diagnostic cast before any abutment crown preparations are made.**

    True/false

13. **Which of the following clinical findings is not a prognostic aid for removable partial denture treatment?**
    A. Patients attitude
    B. Quality of oral hygiene
    C. Exsisting occlusion
    D. Bone index areas

14. **The main reason for mouth preparations for RPD is:**
    A. To create retentive undercuts
    B. To eliminate non-retentive undercuts
    C. To locate survey line
    D. Facilitate placement and removal of prosthesis

15. **The use of occlusal template for evaluating the occlusal plane while planning RPD treatment is done for:**
    A. Location of wear facets
    B. Correction of disharmony between CR and CO
    C. To establish long centric
    D. To identify the location and magnitude of discrepancy in occlusal plane

16. **Treatment of supraerupted maxillary molar which have supraerupted into mandibular edentulous space posterior to which no teeth exist would be?**
    A. Extraction
    B. Enameloplasty
    C. Orthodontic intrusion
    D. None

17 **Which of the following component of RPD framework cause occlusal interferences due to inadequate mouth preparation?**
    A. Proximal guide plane
    B. Rest seat
    C. Denture teeth
    D. Rest

18. **The effectiveness of guide plane is determined by:**
    A. Parallelism
    B. Length/height
    C. Number and position of guide plane
    D. All of the above

NOTES

19. **Guide planes for distal extension prosthesis should be longer than guide plane for tooth supported prosthesis**

    True/False

20. **Crown ledge is a form of lingual ledge rest that is placed in the crown of an abutment tooth. It's function is to:**
    A. Eliminate reciprocal arm
    B. Provide stress equalization
    C. Provide support
    D. Precision guide plane

21. **The height of guide plane adjacent to tooth supported base should be**
    A. 2–4 mm
    B. 1.5 to 2.0 mm
    C. 3 to 6 mm
    D. 8 mm

22. **The lingual guide plane located on the lingual surface of abutment teeth and contacted by major connector are located on:**
    A. Occlusal third
    B. Middle third
    C. Cervical third
    D. Junction of occlusal and middle third

23. **Tooth modifications for alterations in the height of contour is done to**
    A. Determine the path of placement
    B. Modify the retentive undercuts
    C. Provide favourable position for clasp arms
    D. None of the above

24. **Dimpling is a tooth modification procedure. Its main feature is/are**
    A. Enhance retentive undercut
    B. .010 inch undercut at line angle
    C. Parallel to gingival margin
    D. 4 mm mesiodistal and 3 mm occluso gingival in dimension
    E. All of the above

ANSWERS

1 D

2 B Contingency design refers to designing of a removable partial denture prosthesis, so that in the event a questionable tooth is lost a replacement can be conveniently added on to the prosthesis.

3 B Mandibular lingual tori are best treated surgically.

4 A Tuberosity undercuts interferes with proper designing of the prosthesis.

5 C

6 True

7 D

8 D

9 A

10 D

11 A

12 True

13 D

14 D

15 D

16 D When there are no mandibular molars distal to the extruded tooth, the potential for occlusal trauma is not great.

17 D

18 D

19 False

20 D Crown ledge, acts as a precision guide plane when the RPD is fully seated. The crown ledge recess is completely filled by its metal counterpart, which serves to reciprocate the labial retentive clasp arm.

21 A A guide plane adjacent to extension base segment should be 1.5 to 2.0 mm. The reduced height, results in decreased contact of the proximal plate and greater freedom of movement for the RPD.

22 B

23 C

24 E

Support and Impression Procedures for Removable Partial Denture

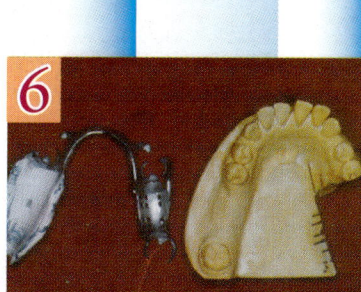

- ❑ Support for the removable partial prosthesis
- ❑ The principle of functional basing
- ❑ Impressions techniques based on physiological basing

SUPPORT FOR THE REMOVABLE PARTIAL PROSTHESIS

Tooth Support

An entirely tooth borne prosthesis is ideal for preservation of remaining oral structures and optimum function.

Composite Support

When complete tooth support is not possible stress should be distributed equally over the remaining natural teeth and alveolar ridge as is the case with distal extension base.

Composite/Tooth-Tissue Support (Fig. 6.1)

i. Unlike periodontal support, the mucosa is resilient, displaceable and can lead to unstable prosthesis.

ii. It is difficult to record the mucosa both at resting (anatomic) and displaced (loaded form) simultaneously.

iii. Distal extension prosthesis under function, compresses the mucosa and acts like a class I lever with the abutment tooth acting as a fulcrum. Thus, it becomes damaging to the abutment tooth with subsequent abutment loss. The solution for distal extension base is:

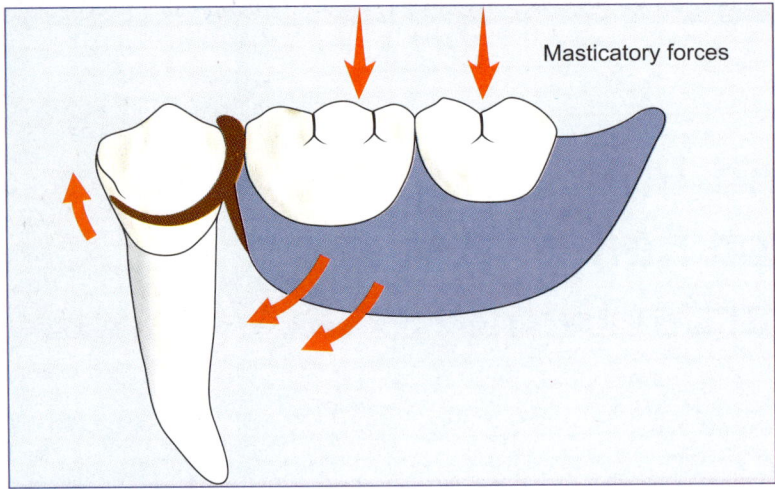

Masticatory forces

To record the functional (placed) form of mucosa and relate it to the abutment tooth so that under loading the prosthesis releases from the abutment tooth without transferring harmful forces. It should be designed to work like a class II lever.

THE PRINCIPLE OF FUNCTIONAL BASING

Functional basing is an attempt to overcome the problem of composite support (tooth-tissue support) in distal extension situation. It is a two-step impression procedure, with two impression materials of differing physical properties.

Purpose

i. The main aim of functional basing is to capture the mucosa in its functional form so that the base can be related to the metal framework in the same relationship that exists between the abutment tooth and the supporting mucosa when occlusal loads are applied.

ii. To accurately extend borders for greater area coverage, so as to reduce stress per unit area of alveolar bone and contribute maximally to the support, stability and retention of the denture.

Indication for Physiologic Basing

- Mandibular distal extension cases, both kennedy Class I and Class II cases.
- Long span anterior edentulous space (at least six anterior teeth missing).

Factors influencing the Support of the Distal Extension Prosthesis (Table 6.1)

Table 6.1	
Factors	*Considerations*
Soft tissue	• Thick and displaceable: Less support • Moderate thickness, firmly attached: Good support • Redundant tissue: surgical removal is advisable, to limit vertical displacement and improve resistance to lateral displacement.
Alveolar bone types	• Cortical bone with rounded contours: Ideal for support, e.g. buccal shelf area • Cancellous bone: Weak bone not good for support • Crest of the alveolar ridge: Should be relieved especially in mandible.
Snow shoe effect	• Broader coverage of residual ridge: Better distribution of load. • Wide denture bases within physiologic limits: Withstands vertical and horizontal forces better.
Impression registration	*Anatomic form*: Is the surface contour of the ridge without occlusal load *Functional form*: Is the surface contour of the ridge under functional/occlusal load. For distal extension bases recording functional form of the ridge is best for support and preservation of abutment teeth.

Framework design considerations	**For distal extension bases**
	i. Use of more anteriorly or mesial occlusal rest is suggested as it
	   • Allows vertical ridge loading
	   • Permits/involves greater ridge area for support.
	   • Transfers stresses to anterior abutments.
	ii. Minor connector contacting the proximal guide plane should get released under occlusal loading of the denture
	iii. Incorporation of indirect retainer to control movement of the prosthesis along the fulcrum axis.
	iv. Incorporation of stress release type of clasps like RPI, RPA, or combination clasp.

Occlusal load	• Reduction in size of occlusal table, and number of artificial teeth • Use of nonanatomic teeth for distal extension bases. • All the above factors determines the occlusal load per unit area of the prosthesis, and enhance longevity of the alveolar bone.

IMPRESSIONS TECHNIQUES BASED ON PHYSIOLOGIC BASING

These are categorized as:
I. Physiologic impression techniques
   i. Mclean-Hindels method
  ii. Functional reline method
 iii. Fluid wax method

II. Selective pressure technique
III. Altered/corrected cast method.

Fluid wax method and selective pressure technique are also referred to as **Corrected Cast method**.

I. Physiologic Impression Technique

Records the ridge portion of the cast in its functional form by placing an occlusal load on the impression tray during the impression procedure.

i. *Mclean-Hindels Technique*

- Records the alveolar ridge in functional form and the remaining natural teeth in anatomic form.
- A custom tray is used to record the alveolar ridge area first followed by picking up the custom tray and remaining teeth in stock tray having hydrocolloid impression material.
- The Hindel's technique differed from Mclean's in that during the pick up stage the hydrocolloid tray had holes for passing fingers in the molar area so as to relate the impression of alveolar ridge to the abutment teeth as it would be under masticatory forces.
- The main disadvantage is that, if the direct retainers are effective then the mucosa over the ridge would always be in functional form and alveolar ridge resorption will occur. If, direct retainers are not effective then due to resiliency of mucosa the denture would be occlusally positioned.

ii. *Functional Reline Method*

- It consists of adding new material to the fitting surface of the denture after processing of the prosthesis at the time of delivery or at a later stage.
- It consist of fabricating the prosthesis on anatomic cast. However, a metal spacer is placed on the cast in the region of alveolar ridge before processing. (Ash No. 7 metal).
- After processing the metal spacer is removed, the denture are functionally relined using low fusing compound and zinc oxide eugenol wash impression material. The denture is processed in acrylic resin and remounted for occlusal corrections before delivery.

- Permanent soft liner (Chair side) like GC soft liner which are silicone based can also be used.

iii. *Fluid Wax Functional Impression*

- It consists of using mouth temperature waxes such as IOWA wax, Korrecta Wax No 4 and Korrecta wax No. 1.
- It requires attaching a custom tray to the framework in the region of extension base. Adequate relief must be provided between the impression tray and the edentulous ridge (1–2 mm).
- Borders of the tray are adjusted up to 2 mm short of the functional limit. Fluid wax is melted and painted at 54°C. Patient is advised to semi-close the mouth and the custom tray with wax painted is placed in patients mouth for 5–7 minutes, for the wax to achieve mouth temperature before it starts flowing.
- A glossy appearance suggest tissue contact is complete.

  Fluid wax may be used to reline an exsisting partial denture or to record the alveolar ridge in functional form
- Fluid wax technique
  - Allows maximum extensions of peripheral borders.
  - Record stress-bearing areas in functional form and non-pressure area in their anatomic form.

II. Selective Pressure Technique

- This technique equalizes the support between the abutment and the soft tissue.
- It consist of directing forces of mastications to those areas of ridge which are best capable of support (primary stress bearing areas).
- The custom tray is selectively relieved by wax spacer. Areas where relief is provided are minimally displaced and in those areas where relief is not provided greater soft tissue displacement occurs.
- Impression materials like zinc oxide-eugenol, rubber base (Polysulfide, poly vinyl siloxane), impression plaster, or fluid wax can be used for selective pressure technique.

III. The Altered Cast/Corrected Cast Method (Figs 6.2A to D)

It consists of 3 main steps:

1. *Acrylic Resin Base Added to the Lattice Work of the Framework*: Resin base is adjusted for extension and border moulding carried out to create a denture border around which the resilient movable tissue can function without discomfort and dislodgement.

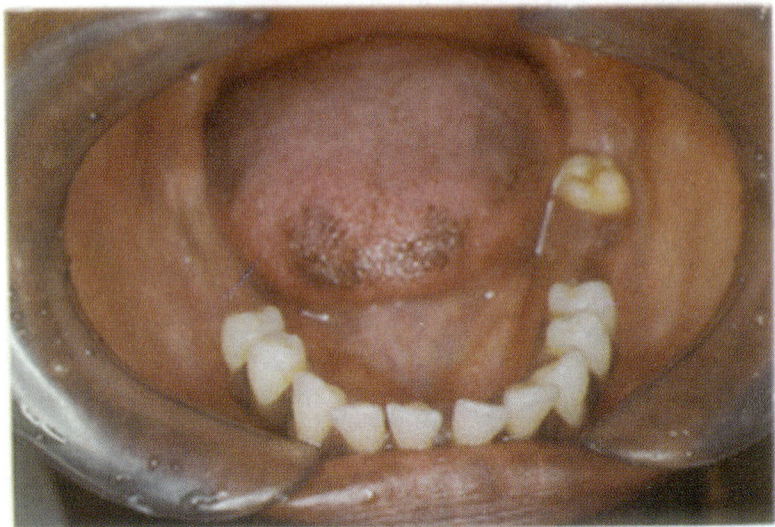

Fig. 6.2A

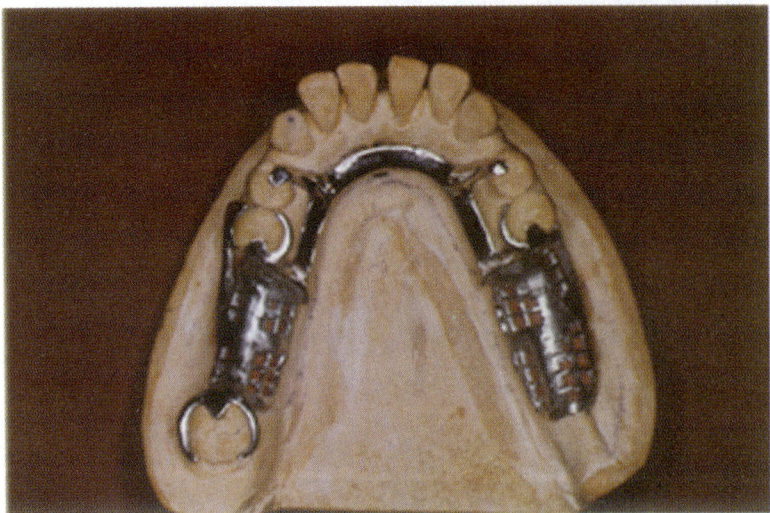

Fig. 6.2B

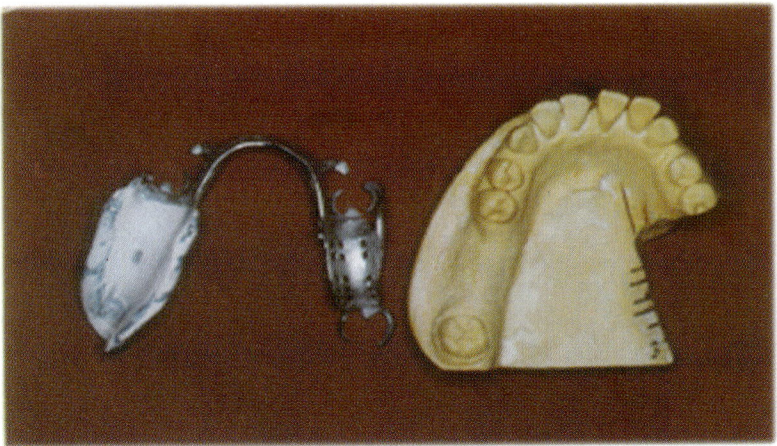

Fig. 6.2C

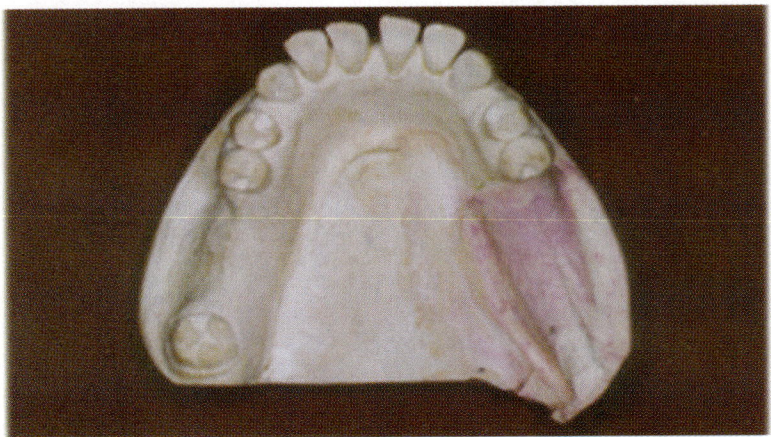

Fig. 6.2D

Figs 6.2 A to D: Fabrication of altered cast

2. *The Final Impression:* It can be registered with fluid wax, zinc-oxide eugenol or rubber base material. After making the final impression the master cast is altered.

3. *Altering the Cast:* The master cast onto which framework was placed after adjustment is now altered by removing the denture bearing area by saw cut 1 mm distal to the terminal abutment. The framework, with final impressions made is now secured to the dentulous portion of the altered master cast and inverted. The area of the impression is now blocked out and poured in different colored stone.

4. The new cast which is obtained by adding the denture-bearing area obtained with functional technique to the

teeth (anatomic) portion of the previous master cast is known as the corrected cast or altered cast.

Need for functional impression

i. Functional impression is required when the underlying mucosa of denture base is displaceable and mucosa is healthy not redundant.

ii. Functional impression should be restricted to situations with uniformly firm ridge consistency so that rebound effect is minimum.

iii. Selective pressure technique can be applied to all varieties of residual ridges as it is customized to mucosal conditions.

iv. Fluid wax and selective pressure techniques are referred to as corrected cast method.

v. Functional reline method is an effective technique which can be carried out for processed denture bases.

vi. Lifting of indirect retainers on finger application of force over the denture base area gives the first visual indication of functional reline for the removable partial denture prosthesis.

MULTIPLE CHOICE QUESTIONS

1. At the time of delivery of processed removable partial denture made for mandibular Kennedy class I situation, lifting of indirect retainers and deviation of jaw on centric closure was observed. What corrections need to be done at the placement procedure.
   A. Functional reline
   B. Altered cast fabrication
   C. Repeat jaw relation record and processing
   D. Functional reline and selective grinding.

2. Functional impression consists of which of the following
   A. Records residual ridge under pressure
   B. Use's displaceable impression material
   C. Records primary stress bearing area in function
   D. Record the ridge under simulated function

3. Which of the following is not the objective of functional impression?
   A. Equalization of tooth and tissue support
   B. Broad stress distribution
   C. Preservation of alveolar ridge
   D. Elimination of need for future relining.

4. Functional impression techniques are primarily indicated for
   A. Bilateral mandibular distal extension situation
   B. Maxillary Class IV situation
   C. Firm mucosal covering distal extension ridges
   D. Long span class III situation

5. Which of the following technique is not a altered cast technique for partial denture impressions?
   A. Selective pressure technique
   B. Fluid wax technique
   C. Corrected cast
   D. Functional reline

6. Dynamic impression making for RPD consists of
   A. Restricted flow of impression material
   B. Selectively relieving displaceable area

C. Application of direct pressure over primary stress area.
D. All of the above
E. None of the above

7. **Which of the following procedure cannot be done at the time of RPD framework delivery?**
   A. Occlusal correction
   B. Adjustment of retentive clasp
   C. Enhancement of denture support
   D. Addition of indirect retention

8. **Fit of removable partial denture base is best evaluated with:**
   A. Disclosing wax
   B. Aerosol spray
   C. Indelible pencil
   D. ZOE paste

9. **For intraoral detection and correction of occlusal discrepancies which of the following is used:**
   A. 21 mm articulating films
   B. Shim stocks
   C. 8 mm articulating films
   D. 14 mm articulating film

10. **Which of the following choice regarding under mentioned statements is true?**

    The best method of removing a wrought wire clasp RPD is by grasping the acrylic-denture bases on each side of the arch. (Statement No. 1).
    The best method of removing a denture with infrabulge clasp is by lifting the approach arm of the clasp assembly. (Statement No. 2)

    A. Both statement 1 and statement 2 are false
    B. Both statement 1 and statement 2 are true
    C. Statement 1 is true, statement 2 in false
    D. Statement 1 is false, statement 2 is true.

11. **Altered cast serves to:**
    A. Relate mucosa to abutment
    B. Relates functional form of ridge to abutment
    C. Relates residual ridge to mucosa
    D. None of the above

12. **Fluid wax technique and functional reline differs in:**
    A. Time of functional loading
    B. Material for functional impression
    C. Method of functional loading
    D. All of the above

13. **Resiliency of periodontal ligament compared to mucosa is:**
    A. 10% less
    B. 20% less
    C. Equal to mucosa
    D. Upto 25% times mucosa is more resilient

14. **Cast partial denture framework can be functionally related to the distal extension base at all stages** *except*:
    A. Before denture delivery
    B. After denture delivery
    C. After framework tryin
    D. Before metal tryin

15. **Mesially placed occlusal rest in RPD design permits all of the following** *except:*
    A. Better utilization of abutment for support
    B. Stress release action
    C. Increased mucosal support
    D. Splinting action on all teeth anterior to rest

16. **The term Realeff was coined by:**
    A. Cummer
    B. Appelgate
    C. Rudolph Hanau
    D. Winkler

17. **Which of the following factors decides the need for functional impression for free end saddle situations?**
    A. Indirect retainers
    B. Index factors
    C. Radiographic evaluation
    D. All of the above

18. **Functional impression provides all of the following effect** *except*:
    A. Support
    B. Stress distribution

NOTES

C. Stress equalization
D. Stress breaker

19. **Dual impression technique for mandibular distal extension bases is must because:**
    A. Support is less
    B. Complicated anatomy due to tongue
    C. Displaceable peripheral tissue
    D. All of the above

20. **Dual impression technique for maxilla is:**
    A. Always needed
    B. Required for long span cases
    C. Rarely indicated
    D. Not required

21. **Primary stress bearing area in a well formed mandibular alveolar ridge is:**
    A. Crest of the ridge
    B. Buccal shelf
    C. Retromolar pad
    D. All of the above

22. **Under-extended impression in tooth borne saddle are:**
    A. Unacceptable
    B. Satisfactory
    C. Unesthetic
    D. Non-functional

23. **Fabrication of tooth-borne partial denture requires which of the following impression form?**
    A. Anatomic form
    B. Functional ridge form
    C. Under extended anatomic impression
    D. Fluid wax

ANSWERS

1 D

2 D Functional impression is a dual impression technique, which consists of recording the residual ridge of a distal extension partial denture under some loading (physiologic pressure) and then relating it to the remainder of the arch (anatomic portion) by means of a secondary impression.

3 D

4 C When mucosal covering over the residual alveolar ridge is firm and uniform, functional impressions are indicated. Firm mucosa, will displace minimum under occlusal loading and hence would have minimum rebound effect. Whenever, residual ridge in distal extension cases is displaceable selective pressure technique are indicated.

5 D Functional reline technique is done for processed denture bases.

6 D Dynamic impression is same as selective pressure technique.

7 D

8 D Disclosing wax is best used for fitting the framework intraorally. Aerosol spray are used for fitting the framework over duplicated master cast before trying it in the patients mouth.

9 B, C Shim stocks helps in verifying the presence and location of occlusal contacts, whereas interferences are identified and marked with articulating film.

10 C

11 C

12 D

13 D

14 D

15 A

16 C

17 D

18 D

19 D

20 C

21 A

22 B

23 A

Laboratory Procedures in Fabrication of Removable Partial Denture Framework

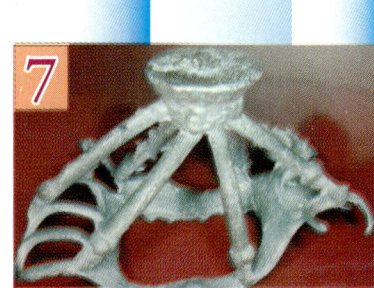

- ❏ Surveying the master cast
- ❏ Duplication of the master cast
- ❏ Wax pattern specifications
- ❏ Waxing, spruing and investing of the partial denture framework
- ❏ Casting of partial denture framework

This chapter primarily discusses only those phases, related to laboratory techniques and materials involved in the fabrication of removable cast partial denture framework. The phases are sequentially discussed as follows:

- I. Surveying the master cast.
- II. Duplication of master cast.
- III. Wax pattern specifications for partial denture components
- IV. Waxing, spruing and investing of the framework
- V. Casting and finishing of the framework.

I. SURVEYING THE MASTER CAST

Designed diagnostic cast should accompany the master cast to the dental laboratory. The master cast is obtained from impression made after all tooth preparations and alterations for receiving cast partial denture framework is complete.

The master cast is surveyed and following observations are made

- i. *Anteroposterior tilt*: Prepared guide planes on the proximal surfaces of abutment teeth determines the correct anterioposterior tilt of the cast.
- ii. *Lateral tilt*: Is determined by that position at which equal retentive undercuts exists on all principal abutments.

165

iii. Checking for any interferences remaining after mouth preparation.

iv. Tripoding/scoring of the master cast for preservation of the tilt of the cast.

v. Locating those areas on the master cast that would need to be blocked out or relieved.

vi. Mark survey line on abutment teeth to delineate the height of contour.

vii. Mark retentive undercuts on the principal abutment teeth in red color to locate the tips of the retentive clasp. The amount of undercut is measured in hundredths of an inch. 0.010 to 0.015 inch undercut are used for short clasp arms whereas 0.015 to 0.020 inch are used for molar clasps.

viii. Mark the rests on the master cast in red.

ix. Transfer the design onto the master cast same as that on the diagnostic cast. Draw the metallic portion in brown color and the acrylic portion in blue.

Block Out and Relief

Block out (wax out): Is the elimination of undesirable undercut areas on the master cast that will be crossed by the rigid parts of the framework.

Types of Blockout and their Indication (Fig. 7.1)

Table 7.1	
Types of block out	*Indications*
Parallel: It extends from the survey line to gingivae	• Beneath minor connector. • Deep interproximal spaces • Soft tissue undercuts beneath major connector. • Undercut areas on teeth to be crossed by the approach arm.
Shaped/ ledging	• Ledging is done on the buccal or lingual surface of teeth to serve as a guide for accurate placement of clasp arm. • Most commonly shaped block out is done in the region of clasp tip only
Arbitrary	• Arbitrary block out is done on those areas of the master cast which lies outside the design area. It is done to facilitate withdrawal of the blocked out cast from the duplicating material.
Relief	• It is done to create a space between the framework and the cast or soft tissue. • It is given beneath mandibular major connectors always.
	• It is done over edentulous ridge area beneath the framework extension to provide attachment for the acrylic resin and to form internal finish lines.

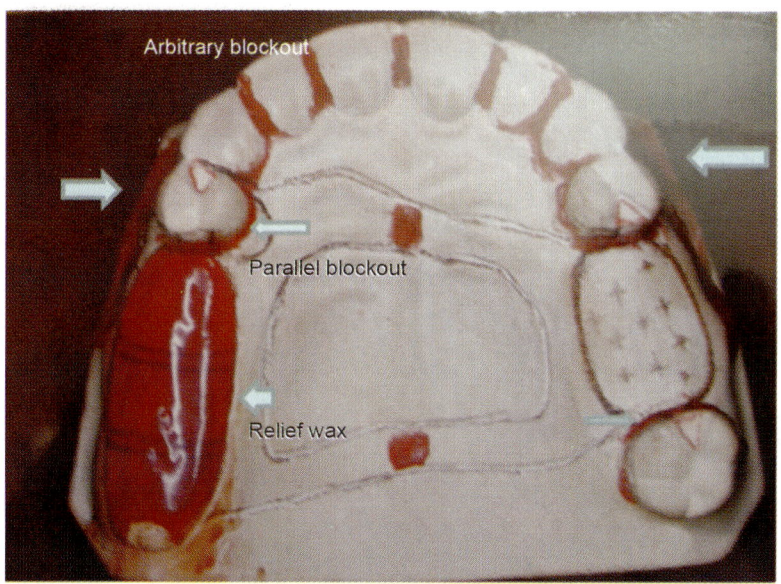

Arbitrary blockout

Parallel blockout

Relief wax

Fig. 7.1: Different types of wax blockout and relief

II. DUPLICATION OF THE MASTER CAST (Fig. 7.2)

Duplication of the master cast is done after completion of block out and relief.

It is done to produce a copy of the master cast in invest-ment material or to obtain a refractory cast.

A refractory cast for partial denture is made up of phos-phate bonded investment material which is capable of with-standing high temperatures without disintegrating and also undergoes expansion to compensate for metal shrinkage.

Duplicating Materials

Reversible hydrocolloid (Agar Agar) is most commonly used for duplication. Alginate irreversible hydrocolloid may also be used by increasing the volume of water up to 3 times the volume used for a regular impression.

The other material which can be used for duplication is silicone based polyvinyl chloride. Agar Agar is commonly used as it can be reused and is economical.

The blocked out master cast are placed in a duplicating flask, which is used to support the cast and confine the hydrocolloid since it aids in controlling shrinkage. The Agar Agar solution is poured into the duplicating flask at 57° to 60° C. The refractory cast, is obtained by pouring investment material into the mould obtained by duplica-tion of the master cast.

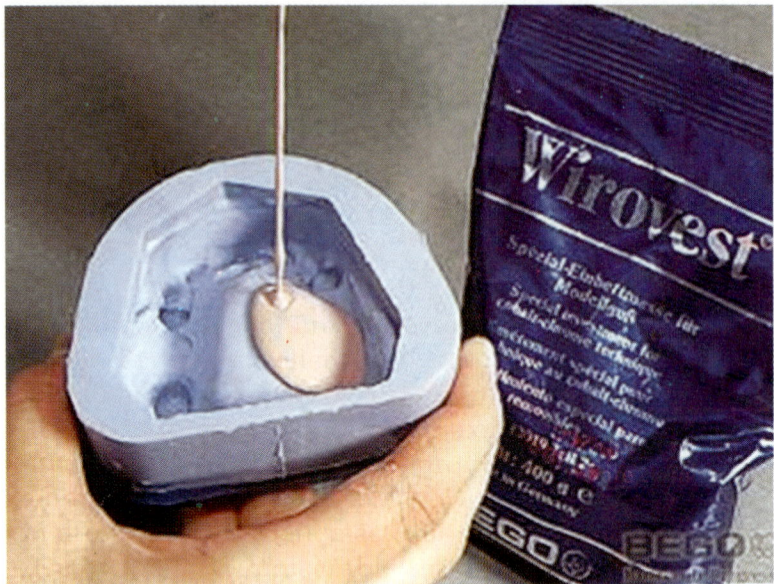

Fig. 7.2: Duplication of master cast

Treating the Refractory Cast

The surface of the refractory cast when set is treated with either model spray or wax. It helps to make the cast less susceptible to abrasion and ensures a smooth dense surface for waxing of the framework.

Refractory cast is heated in hot air oven for about 1 hour up to 200° C before either application of model spray or bees wax. Such a treatment further helps in sticking of the wax pattern to the cast.

III. WAX PATTERN SPECIFICATIONS FOR PARTIAL DENTURE COMPONENTS (Table 7.2)

See next page for Table 7.2.

IV. WAXING, SPRUING AND INVESTING OF THE PARTIAL DENTURE FRAMEWORK (Figs 7. 3A and B)

Spruing

The sprue provides a channel for the flow of molten alloy. It leads the molten metal from the crucible into the mold cavity. It also provides a reservoir of molten metal to continue to feed the mold cavity during the solidification process thereby compensating for casting shrinkage.

	Table 7.2	
	Component	*Wax gauge*
1.	**Direct Retainers** • Retentive arm of combination clasp • Aker's clasp • Cast circumferential clasp • Bar type clasp • Reciprocal arm	18 gauge round wax 12 gauge 12 gauge half round wax 12 gauge half round wax 12 gauge half round for premolars. 8 gauge half round for molars.
2.	**Major Connectors**	
	• Mandibular linguoplate	Inferior border 6 gauge half pear shaped wax form, reinforced with 24 gauge sheet wax. Superior apron is of 24 gauge sheet wax.
	• Mandibular lingual bar with continuous bar retainer	Inferior portion 6 gauge half round wax, for the lingual bar. Continuous bar retainer pattern formed by adapting two strips (3 mm wide) of 28 gauge sheet wax over the cingula and into interproximal embrasure.
	• Labial bar	6 gauge half pear shaped wax form reinforced with 22–24 gauge sheet wax or similar plastic pattern.
	• Lingual bar	6 gauge half pear shaped wax form reinforced with 22–24 gauge sheet wax.
	• Single palatal strap	Anatomic replica pattern equivalent to 22–24 gauge wax type depending upon the arch width.
	• Single broad palatal connector	24 gauge sheet wax thickness or equivalent anatomica pattern.
	• Anterior posterior strap	Anterior strap 8 to 10 mm wide anterior replica pattern of 22 gauge wax thickness.
	• Posterior palatal component	Half oval in form of 6 gauge wax thickness and width
	• Complete palatal coverage	Anatomic replica pattern equivalent to 22–24 gauge wax thickness.
3	**Proximal plate**	8 gauge half round wax on the prepared guide plane.
4	**Minor connector** • Joining occlusal rest to major connector	10 gauge round wax.
5	**Tooth bound saddle**	2 sheet of 24 gauge casting wax, joined at the crest and metal base trimmed 0.5 mm inferior to the penciled outline of the framework.
6	**Occlusal rest**	10 gauge round wax form.
7	**Minor connector:** Covering edentulous ridge for resin retention.	2 parallel pieces of 12 gauge half round wax connected with cross rugs to form a ladder like pattern.
8	**Relief for denture base**	20 gauge wax sheet.
9	**Relief-over:** Median palatine raphe, tori or underneath lingual bar/plate.	32 gauge sheet wax.

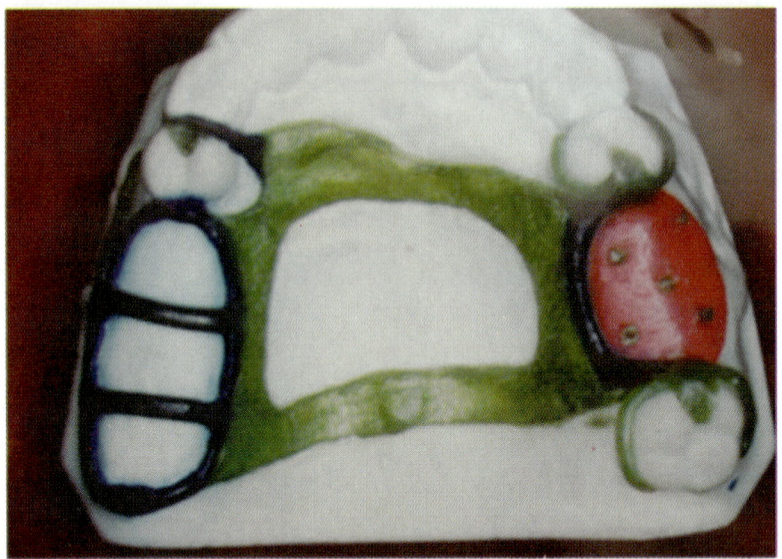

Fig. 7.3A

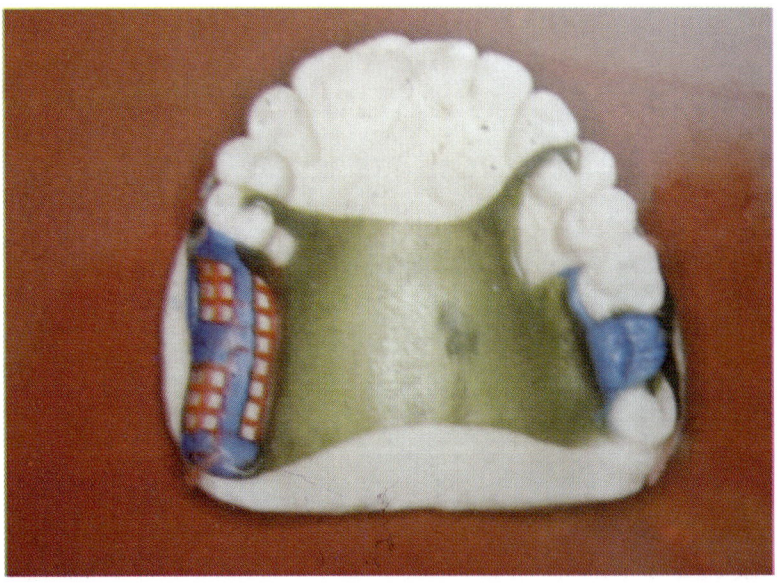

Fig. 7.3B

Figs 7.3A and B: Waxed-up refractory cast ready for spruing

Principles and Requirement of Spruing

i. Sprue should be large enough to feed the metal into mold cavity without freezing the metal.

ii. The sprues should be direct in approach to the mold cavity and induce minimum turbulence in the stream of molten metal.

iii. Main sprue should always be attached to the bulkier section of the wax pattern.

iv. Accessory sprues should be attached to thinner section for completeness of the casting.

v. Sprue channel should originate from a common point in the crucible, and its point of attachment to the wax pattern must be flared.

Types of Spruing (Figs 7.4A and B)

A. According to location of main sprue
1. Direct
2. Indirect
3. Rear.

B. According to the number of sprue
1. Single
2. Multiple.

According to the Location of Main Sprue

• **Direct or top spruing:** It is done for majority of the maxillary cases. It consists of the sprue originating from top of the wax pattern from the crucible former.

• **Indirect/bottom spruing:** Mandibular partial dentures are usually sprued through a hole in the center of the refractory cast. It consists of a 7 mm wide and about 10 mm long central sprue coming out of the central hole. Main and auxilliary sprues are attached to the central sprue approximately 7 mm below the tip of central sprue.

The main advantage of indirect spruing is that the initial thrust of molten metal is directed against the tip of the central sprue and the resulting turbulence and impurities are confined to the central sprue rather than being distributed to the main sprue.

• **Rear Spruing:** It consists of a single large sprue attached to the back end of the maxillary major connector. It is mostly used with complete cast palatal major connector.

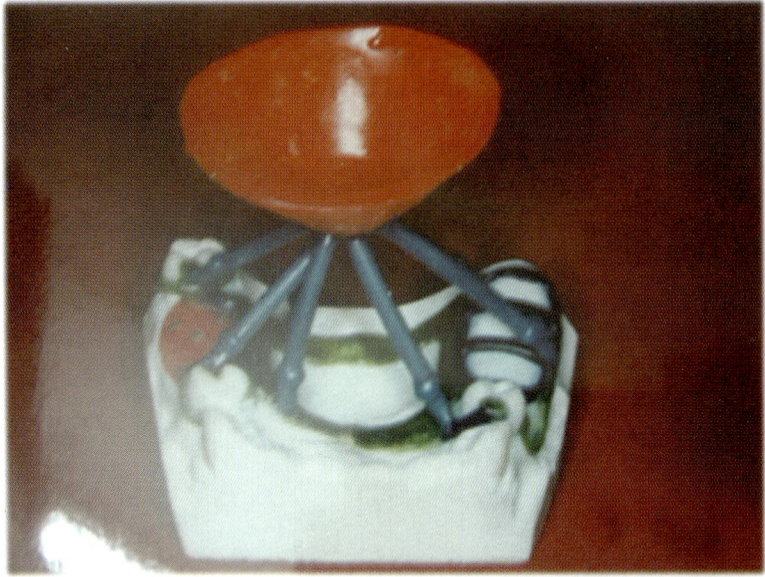

Fig. 7.4A: Direct spruing

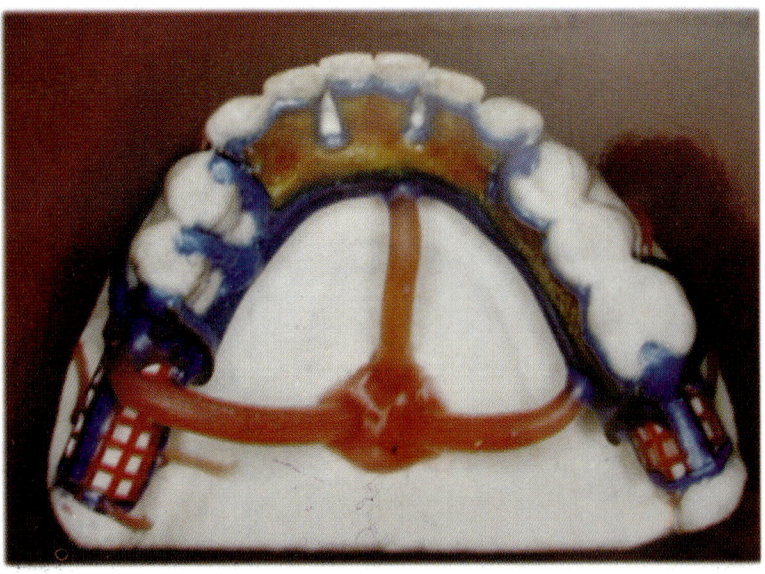

Fig. 7.4B: Indirect spruing

Figs 7.4A and B: Different types of spruing (Direct and indirect)

According to the Number of Sprues

- **Single spruing:** It consists of using a single sprue as in complete cast palate and cast metal bases for the mandibular arch.

- **Multiple spruing:** It consists of main sprue of 8 to 12 gauge round wax shapes and 12 to 18 gauge round wax auxilliary sprues.

Investing the Sprued Wax Pattern

Investment material is applied in two separate steps. The first is a thin coat called paint on investment which is applied with a brush to ensure that air is not trapped adjacent to the pattern. The second or the outer investment is poured or vibrated into the investment ring around the pattern and cast after the paint on investment has set.

The purpose of the investment is as follows:
1. To provide strength necessary to resist the forces created by the stream of molten metal.
2. To make a smooth surface for the mold cavity so the casting will require as little finishing as possible.
3. To establish an avenue of escape for most of the gases created by the burnout and casting procedure.
4. To compensate for some of the dimensional changes of the metal when it goes from the molten to the solid state.

BURNOUT, CASTING AND FINISHING OF THE FRAMEWORK (Fig. 7.5)

Purpose of Burnout

- Dries the moisture out of the mold.

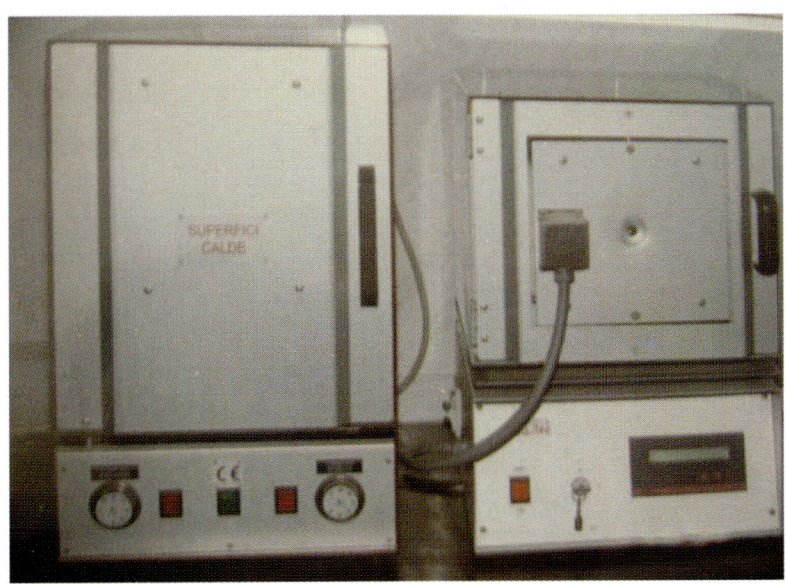

Fig. 7.5: Burnout oven and thermal microprocessor for heating the refractory cast

- Eliminates plastic and wax pattern.
- Expands the mold to compensate for shrinkage of the metal.
- Complete removal of carbon residue from the interstices of investment material.

V. CASTING OF PARTIAL DENTURE FRAMEWORK (Fig. 7.6)

The casting of partial denture framework varies with alloy and technique used. All methods uses force to quickly inject the molten metal into the mold cavity. The type of force used for injecting the alloy could be either centrifugal, or air pressure under vaccum. Adequate force should be used to ensure completeness of the casting.

For melting of alloy either gas-oxygen blowtorch, acetylene, electric conduction or induction method may be used.

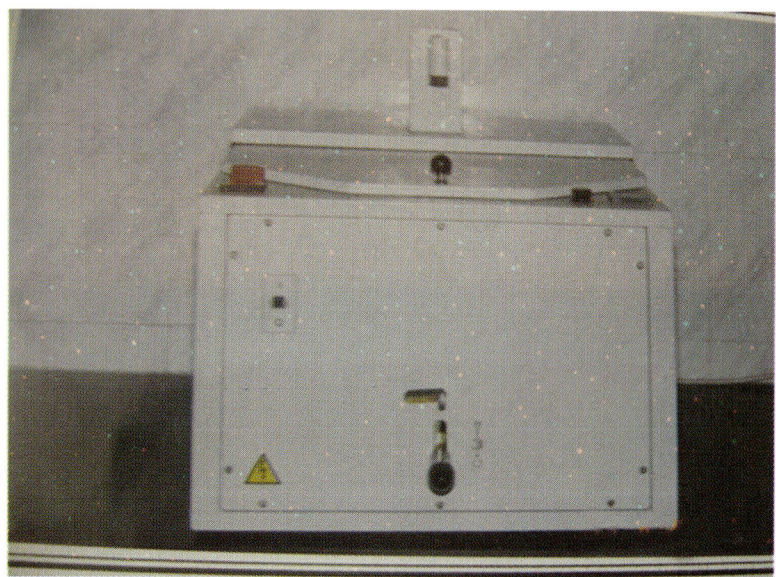

Fig. 7.6: Induction casting machine

Recovery of the Casting

Gold Alloy

Quenching the casting in water after allowing the mold to bench cool for 12 minutes is ideal for gold alloy and is known as the softening heat treatment. Softening, heat treatment of gold is done for the purpose of easier finishing.

Hardening Heat Treatment

Before polishing the gold framework it is placed in an oven that has been heated to 450° C and allowed to cool to 250° C over 30 minutes after which it is removed from the furnance and bench cooled.

Gold alloys are also always pickled in an acidic solution to remove metal deposits, oxidation products and contaminants.

Cobalt-Chromium Alloy (Fig. 7.7)

These are usually allowed to bench cool and divested. They are not cleaned by pickling. Finishing and polishing of the framework is done with high speed equipments. Gross finishing is done with abrasive stones or sintered diamonds. Chromium cobalt castings are electropolished (controlled depletion of metal) before final polishing with rubber points.

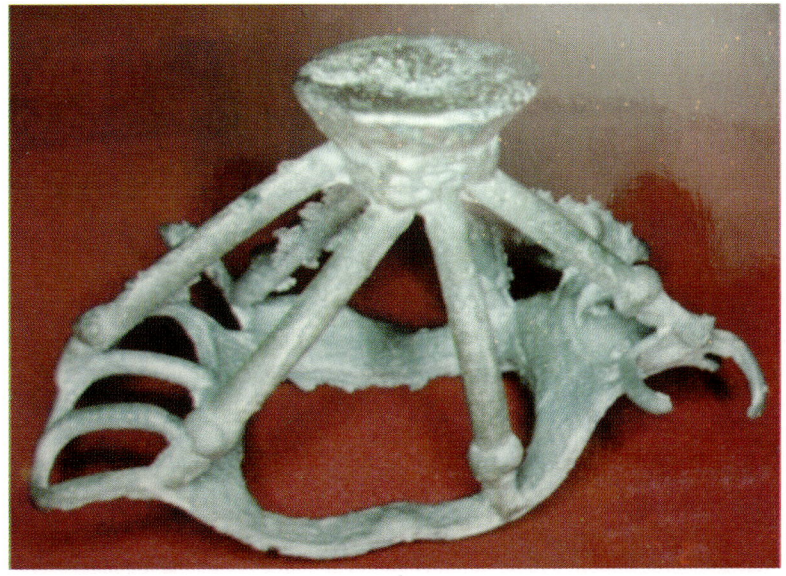

Fig. 7.7: Divested cobalt-chromium casting

MULTIPLE CHOICE QUESTIONS

1. **While designing a removable partial denture framework which of the following is not true?**
   A. Dentist should survey the diagnostic cast
   B. Dentist should draw the design on the definitive cast
   C. The laboratory personal should draw the design on both the casts
   D. None of the above

2. **Which of the following is not true for tripoding the partial denture cast?**
   A. Tripoding preserves the tilt of the cast
   B. Tripoding is done at the selected path of placement
   C. Tripode marks are 3 widely separated points in different plane
   D. Tripoding is done on those areas of the cast not included in the design

3. **Internal finish line is not required for which of the following situations?**
   A. Metal bases
   B. Kennedy class III situations
   C. Nail head retention
   D. All of the above

4. **Ledging on the abutment tooth is done for:**
   A. Location of retentive undercut
   B. Location of reciprocal arm
   C. Precise retentive tip placement
   D. Blocking out non-critical undercuts

5. **Which of the following procedure is not done before duplication of the master cast?**
   A. Block out and relief
   B. Wetting of cast with slurry water
   C. Application of cast sealer over the design
   D. Model spraying of the cast

6. **The rate of stone cast solubility in tap water is:**
   A. 1 part of stone in 500 parts of water
   B. 1 part of stone in 200 parts of water
   C. 1 part of stone in 800 parts of water
   D. 1 part of stone in 600 parts of water

7. **Arbitrary block out is done on the master cast. The main reason behind the block out is:**
   A. To prevent distortion of the duplicating material
   B. To facilitate removal of the stone cast
   C. To prevent tearing of the duplicating material.
   D. All of the above

8. **Which of the following is used for mixing investment mix?**
   A. Tap water
   B. Boiled water
   C. Filter water
   D. Modelling liquid

9. **Which of the following is the reason for duplication of master cast during fabrication of cast partial denture?**
   A. Fitting of removable partial denture framework
   B. Processing a temporary prosthesis
   C. Fabrication of an investment cast
   D. All of the above

10. **The refractory cast on which the pattern for cast partial denture framework will be placed should be oven dried at 93° C for 1 hour in an ventend oven:**

    True/False

11. **Wrought wire retainer can be added to the cast partial denture framework by which of the following technique?**
    A. Electric soldering
    B. Cold welding
    C. Centrifugal casting
    D. All of the above

12. **Which of the following is the first procedure/step after waxing the investment cast?**
    A. Spraying surface tension reducer
    B. Application of bees wax dip
    C. Paint on investment
    D. Spruing the wax pattern

13. **The reason for doing ringless casting for Cobalt-Chromium alloy framework is:**
    A. To allow for greater mold expansion
    B. To save time
    C. To achieve uniform expansion.

NOTES

14. **Function of burnout process before casting is to:**
    A. Drive off the moisture
    B. Vaporizes and eliminate the pattern
    C. Compensate for metal shrinkage on cooling
    D. All of the above

15. **Casting shrinkage of gold and cobalt-chromium alloy is respectively:**
    A. 1.74%, 2.3%
    B. 1.2%, 2.3%
    C. 1.0%, 2.0%
    D. None of the above

16. **The powder to liquid ratio for paint on investment mix should be different from that of refractory cast.**

    True/False

17. **For divesting of casted framework 50 mm grit aluminium oxide is used. The correct pressure and the distance of the nozzle delivering oxide from the framework should be:**
    A. 5000 psi, 2 cm
    B. 8000 psi, 4 cm
    C. 2000 psi, 1 inch
    D. 1000psi, 6 inch

18. **For final polishing and luster of the metal framework which of the following is used?**
    A. Prophy paste
    B. Tripoli
    C. Hydrochloric acid
    D. Green soap and ammonia solution

ANSWERS

1 B The dentist should mark only the diagnostic cast.

2 C

3 D

4 C

5 D Model spraying is done to the refractory cast. Also, the design over the master cast should be covered with a light coat of cast sealer to maintain the design.

6 A Cast should be wetted in slurry water before duplication. Leave the casts in slurry water no longer than is necessary to thoroughly wet them.

7 D

8 D

9 D

10 True

11 A

12 D

13 A

14 D

15 A

16 True

The mix for paint on investment should have 1 ml more liquid for the same amount of investment powder.

The reason is that:

- It allows better adaptation of investment to the wax pattern.
- Permits escapement of the gases formed during burnout
- It allows less expansion of the outer investment layer than the cast and eliminate the formation of fins.

17 D

18 D

Planning Occlusal Relationship for Removable Partial Denture

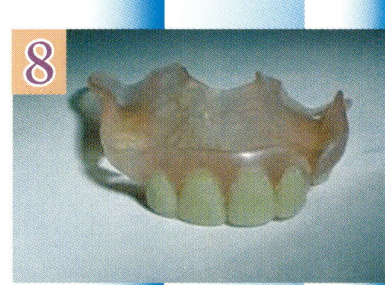

- ❑ Maxillomandibular positions and occlusion in removable partial denture
- ❑ Desirable occlusion contact for removable partial denture situations
- ❑ Methods for establishing occlusal relationship for removable partial denture

In establishing occlusion on a removable partial denture, the occlusion of the remaining natural teeth dictates the occlusion of the prosthesis.

The key in deciding what position (Centric Relation or Centric Occlusion) to restore the occlusion of a removable partial denture, depends on which is the most reproducible position for the individual patient. Satisfactory occlusion for removable partial denture patient should include the following (Fig. 8.1):

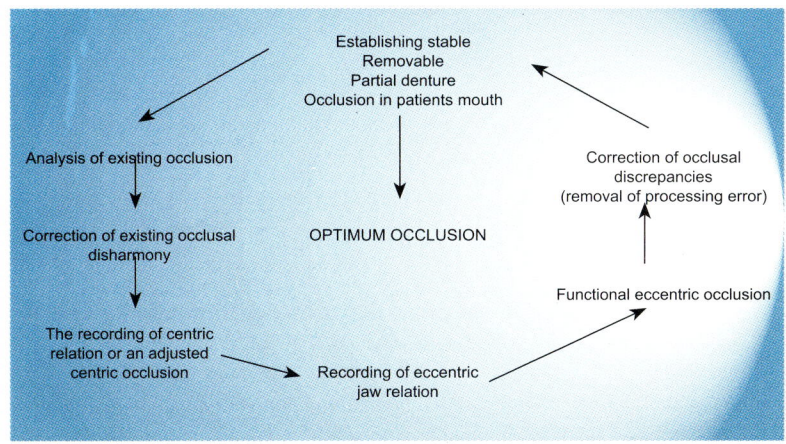

Fig. 8.1: Establishing optimum Occlusion on RPD

Maxillomandibular Positions and Occlusion in Removable Partial Denture

		Indication in Removable Partial Denture
1.	**Centric Occlusion**	i. Stable, maximal occlusal contacts in centric occlusion exists when sufficient number of posterior teeth remains and provides positive occlusal positioning of the mandible at an acceptable vertical dimension.
		ii. No pathosis exists at centric occlusion (no excessive tooth wear, medio lateral slides, widening of periodontal ligaments or tooth mobility exist).
		iii. Indicated for Kennedy class III, class IV and some class II.
2.	**Centric Relation**	i. When there are insufficient occlusal contacts present to provide for a stable mandibular occlusal position.
		ii. When eccentric contacts are desired on the prosthesis.
		iii. When a removable partial denture opposes a maxillary or mandibular complete denture.
		iv. Kennedy class I, and most class II removable partial dentures.
3.	**Long centric/ freedom in centric**	i. Allows a small area 1–1.5 mm on which bilateral stable occlusal contacts can occur simultaneously.
		ii. There is freedom of movement from centric relation to centric Occlusion. The muscular activity is minimum and mandible is positioned in a stable unrestricted position.

Desirable Occlusal Contact for Removable Partial Denture Situations

1.	Bilateral simultaneous contact	Regardless of maxillomandibular position, the opposing posterior teeth (natural and artificial) must contact simultaneously on both side.
2.	Tooth supported/Kennedy class III partial denture	Occlusal contact should follow that on remaining natural teeth present if the vertical dimension of occlusion is not to be altered.
3.	Maxillary complete denture against mandibular distal extension partial denture	Eccentric bilateral balanced contacts is must. Also, opposing protrusive balance required for effective distribution of stresses
4.	Mandibular class I and II removable partial denture against natural teeth	Working side eccentric contacts only
5.	Maxillary class I removable partial denture against natural teeth	Bilateral balanced occlusal contacts are must
6.	Maxillary and mandibular class II situation against each other	Working side contacts only
7.	Kennedy Class IV removable partial denture	Maxillary and mandibular anteriors must contact in occlusion or centric relation.
8.	Contacts at raised vertical dimension of occlusion	Whenever vertical dimension of occlusion of patient is altered with removable partial denture, remaining natural teeth should also be modified with cast restorations or by overlaying the occlusal surfaces of the natural teeth with the removable partial denture framework.

Methods for Establishing Occlusal Relationship for Removable Partial Denture

1.	Direct apposition	• This method is used when sufficient number of teeth remains for establishing satisfactory relationship. When, few teeth are to be replaced on short denture bases and there are no occlusal abnormalities present.
2.	Inter occlusal record with posterior teeth remaining	• It is used when sufficient natural teeth remains to support but the relation of opposing natural teeth does not permit hand articulation. Metal reinforced wax is used for recording Centric occlusion or centric relation position, e.g. aluwax. Wax record should not contact the mucosa and is further corrected by free flowing metal oxide paste.
3.	Occlusal relation using occlusion rims on record bases	• This method is used with distal extension bases or when a large tooth-supported space is present. • It consists of stable resin base with occlusal wax rims in the area of missing teeth. • Occlusion rims substitute for missing posterior teeth and provide support for inter occlusal record. • Quick setting impression plaster or bite registration paste can be used for making inter occlusal record.
4.	Jaw relations entirely on occlusion rims	• This method is used when there are no remaining natural teeth posteriorly as in maxillary complete denture opposed by mandibular distal extensions or maxillary and mandibular Kennedy class I against each other.
5.	Jaw relation established by registering occlusal pathways or functionally generated pathways	• It records functional pathways and uses occluding template rather than a cast of opposing arch for teeth arrangement. • It requires complete rehabilitation of intact opposing arch against which the removable partial denture can be fabricated. • The partially edentulous arch in which removable partial denture is to be fabricated, hard inlay wax is placed over the stable denture base and patient is asked to carry out all extremes of mandibular movements. The intact arch, generates indentations in the inlay wax which is later poured in stone and a occlusal template obtained, against which artificial teeth of removable partial denture are arranged. Advantages of functionally generated path techniques are as follows: • Harmonious occlusion. • No recording of complex mandibular movements required. • Recovery of lost vertical dimension of occlusion. • Errors in occlusion are minimized. • Eliminates the need of articulator

MULTIPLE CHOICE QUESTIONS

1. **Bilateral balanced occlusion is advocated in:**
   A. Tooth supported RPD's
   B. Mandibular class II RPD against maxillary natural dentition
   C. Mandibular class I RPD against maxillary natural dentition
   D. Maxillary class I RPD against mandibular class I RPD.

2. **Balanced occlusion is not present in:**
   A. Natural dentition
   B. Complete denture
   C. Full mouth rehabilitation
   D. Removable partial denture

3. **Hand articulation is best done for**
   A. Short span class III RPD
   B. Fixed partial denture replacing single tooth
   C. Class IV RPD
   D. All of the above

4. **Which of the following occlusal surfaces are best suited against natural dentition?**
   A. Resin
   B. Gold
   C. Porcelain
   D. Resin teeth with gold occlusal surface

5 **Which of the following cast is used for recording jaw relations in a distal extension situation in a mandibular jaw?**
   A. Diagnostic cast
   B. Master cast
   C. Refractory cast
   D. Functional cast

6. **Choice of artificial teeth against complete denture with dental porcelain denture teeth would be:**
   A. Acrylic resin
   B. Gold occlusal surfaces
   C. Porcelain teeth
   D. None of the above

7. **Regarding functionally generated path technique for artificial teeth arrangement in RPD, which of the following is true:**
   A. Eliminates the need for an articulator
   B. Teeth arrangement is done against functionally generated occlusal template
   C. Ensures complete harmony
   D. All of the above

8. **What type of occlusal contacts are desired for unilateral distal extension RPD?**
   A. Bilateral balance
   B. Unilateral balance
   C. Canine guidance
   D. Centric occlusion

9. **Contact of mandibular anteriors with maxillary anteriors should be avoided in denture patients. However, in which of the following situations mandibular anteriors should contact maxillary anteriors?**
   A. Maxillary class IV RPD against mandibular natural teeth
   B. Maxillary denture against mandibular natural teeth
   C. Maxillary denture against mandibular denture.
   D. All of the above

NOTES

ANSWERS

1 D
2 A
3 D
4 D
5 D
6 C
7 D
8 B
9 A

NOTES

Suggested Reading

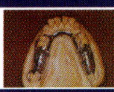

1. Treatment of Partially Edentulous Patients: Louis J Boucher , Robert P. Renner .The C.V Mosby Company. ST. Louis. Toronto, LONDON. 1982.
2. Removable Partial Prosthodontics – Ernest L. Miller 1972 The Williams & Wilkins Company, Baltimore.
3. Dental Laboratory Procedures ~Removable Partial Dentures, Vol: 3; The C.V Mosby Company, Kenneth D. RUDD, Robert M, Morrow; Harlod F. Eissman.
4. Partial Dentures – George Alexander Lammie, W.R.E Laird, Fifth Edition; Blackwell Scientific Publication, Oxford, London.
5. McCracken's. Removable Partial. Prosthodontics. Glen P. McGivney and Alan B. Carr, 10th edition. Mosby,. Inc, St. Louis.
6. Stewart's Clinical Removable Partial Prosthodontics 3rd Ed. Quintessence, 2003.

NOTES

References

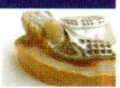

1. Aviv/Z.Ben-Ur et al: RLS – the lingually retained clasp assembly for distal extension removable partial dentures. Quintessence International. 1990;21(3):221–3.

2. A.J Levis and T.G Goodall – Duplication variables related to partial denture castings. Aust. Dental journal . 1977;(22)6:478–80.

3. AG Wegner, Frank C Traweek: Comparison of major connectors for removable partial dentures. JPD 1982;47:243–5.

4. Brian D. Monteith – Management of loading forces on mandibular distal extension prosthesis. Part I ; Evaluation of concepts of design. JPD 1984; 52(5):73–681.

5. Bert T Cecconi, Kamal Asgar, Edward Dootz – Removable partial denture abutment tooth movement as affected by inclination of residual ridges and type of loading. JPD 1971;(25)4:375–381.

6. Bennie S. Dukes Hubert Fields – Comparison of disclosing media used for adjustment of removable partial denture frameworks. JPD 1981;45(4):380–82.

7. Celia Y I, Jack DP – Cobalt Chromium – Titanium alloy for Removable partial dentures. The Int Journal of Prosthodontics; 1997;10(4):309–17.

8. David N Fritell *et al*: Laboratory accuracy in casting removable partial denture frameworks. *JPD* 1985;54(4);856–62.

9. David Benson and Vladimir W. S – A clinical evaluation of removable partial dentures with I – bar retainers. Part I ; JPD March 1979; (41)3:246–54.

10. Ernest L. Miller: Systems for classifying partially dentulous arches. JPD. 1970;24(1):25–40.

11. Ejvind Budtz – Jorgensen and Gilbert Bochet – Alternate framework design for removable partial dentures. JPD 1998;(80)1:58–65.

12. Frank R. Lauciello – Technique for remounting removable partial dentures opposing maxillary complete dentures. JPD 1981; Vol 45(3):336–40.

13. Frank J. Kratochvil – Maintaining supporting structures with a removable partial prosthesis. JPD. 1971;25(2):167–74.

14. George W. Hindels – Load distribution in extension saddle partial dentures. JPD 2001; 85(4):324–48.

15. Gus J. Livaditis – Indexing procedures for converting removable partial dentures after extractions while the patient retains the prosthesis. JPD. 1999; 81(4): 485–91.

16. Herman B Dumbrigue, JF Esquivel: Selective pressure single impression procedure for tooth-mucosa-supported removable partial dentures. JPD. 1993;80(2):259–61.

17. Ira D. Zinner – Semiprecision rest system for distal – extension removable partial dentures. JPD 1979;(42)1:4–11.

18. JC Davenport, et al: Indirect retention. BDJ, 2001;190(3):128–32.

19. James S Brudvik, David Reimers: The tooth removable partial denture interface. *JPD* 1992;68(6):924–27.

20. JD Browning, LW Meadors, JD Eick – Movement of three removable partial denture clasp assemblies under occlusal loading. JPD 1986; 55(1):69–74.

21. John W.Mc Cartney: Lingual plating for reciprocation. JPD Dec 1979; 42(6) 624–25.

22. JC Davenport et al: Tooth preparation. BDJ, 2001;190(6):288–94.

23. J Peitrokovski, Chapman – The form of the mandibular anterior lingual alveolar process in partially edentulous patients. JPD 1981;45(4):371–75.

24. JT Bridgeman, et al: Comparison of Titanium and Cobalt Chromium removable partial denture clasps. JPD. 1997;178: 187–193.

25. KK Kapur, *et al*: A randomised clinical trial of two basic removable partial denture designs. Part II Comparisons of masticatory scores. JPD 1977;78(1):15–21.

26. M.I Mac Entec – Biologic sequelae of tooth replacement with removable partial dentures: A case for caution. JPD. 1993;70: 132–134.

27. Mitchell A Stern, James S Brudvik, R. Frank: Clinical evaluation of removable partial denture rest seat adaptation. JPD 1985;53(5):658–62.

28. N Wakabayashi: A short tern clinical follow up study of superplastic titanium alloy for major connectors of removable partial dentures. JPD 1997;77(6)583–87.

29. Richard P Frank, J Nicholls – An investigation of the effectiveness of indirect retainers. JPD 1977;38(5):494–506.

30. Roy Storer—Partial denture saddle correction. BDJ1962;5:454–59.

31. Randa Diwan, *et al*: Pattern waxes and inaccuracies in fixed and removable partial denture castings. JPD 1997;77(5):553–55.

32. U Santana, Penin *et al*: An accurate method for occlusal registration and altered-cast impression for removable partial dentures during the same visit as the framework tryin. *JPD* 1998; 80(5): 615–18.

33. Yoshiaki Taga et al – New method for divesting cobalt-chromium alloy casting. Sandblasting with a mixed abrasive powder. *JPD* 2001; 85(4):357–362.

34. The Dental Clinics of North America-Symposium on Prosthodontics – Charles L Bolender 1970;14(3).

❑❑❑

Index

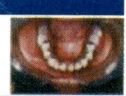

All acrylic partial denture 03, 33
    flexible partial denture (Dental d, Valplast) 06
    overlay 03
    splint 03
Altered cast 11
Andrews bridge 12
Applegate rules (Table 1.2) 10
Augmentative, regenerative therapy 03

Biomechanics 109
    lever action 109
Blockout relief 164
    arbitrary 164
    ledging (Table 7.1),164
Bone index area 137
    negative factor (Table 5.1)137
    positive factor (Table 5.1) 137
Burnout oven 171
    thermal microprocessor (Fig 7.5),171
Cast 165
    Refractory 165
Cast partial denture 04
    metallic denture
      (gold, base metal, titanium alloy) 06
    parts of 04,05
Casting 173
    recovery of 174
Centric relation 181
    centric occlusion 181
    long centric 182
    functionally generated 183
Circumferential clasp 68
    (ring clasp, embrasure clasp, half and half clasp,
    reverse action clasp) 69,70,71
Clasp assembly 12
    classification of 67
    requirements for 63
    retentive clasp 15
Clasp position 113
    quadrilateral design 113
    tripodal design 113
Combination clasp 12
Combination syndrome 12
Complete dentures 17
Complete palatal coverage 26
Cross arch stabilization and bracing 03

Dental implants 02
Denture base 95
Denture teeth 95
    cross-linked acrylic resin (Table 2.10) 97
    porcelain 97
    tube teeth 98
Direct retainer 60
    parts of 62
    purpose 60
    types (intracoronal, extracoronal) 60
Distal extension 02,110
    extension based denture 13
Dual support 03
Duplication 166
    duplicating materials 167
    reversible hydrocolloid (agar-agar) 167
    alginate 167

Esthetics 02, 03
Every denture 34

Finish lines 45
    external finish lines 45
    internal finish lines 46
Fixed partial dentures 02
Food impaction 134
    Horizontal (Table 5.1) 134
    Vertical (table 5.1) 134
Fulcrum line 13
    retentive fulcrum line 15
Functional impression 112
    functional basing 150
Functional reline 112, 151

Gillett bridge 13
Guide planes 123

Heat treatment 174
    hardening 174

Impression 151
    Techniques for 153
    registration of anatomic/functional form 151
    physiologic impression 154
    fluid wax (Iowa/Korecta wax no.4) 152
Indirect retainers 86
    rationale 86
    guidelines 88
    functions 88
    form of 88

Interferences 124
    hard tissue 126
    soft tissue 126

Kennedy's bar 29

Labial bar 30
Laboratory procedures,165
Lingual bar 29
Linguoplate 29
Long edentulous span 03

Major connector 23
    classification 23
    functions 23
    requirements and characteristics 24
Maxillofacial defects 04
    acquired 04
    congenital 04
Maxillomandibular relationship 03
    vertical dimension of occlusion 04
Milling 13
Minor connector 42
    functions 42
    location and types (Table 2.5) 42
    design considerations (Fig. 2.8) 43
Model spray 168
Mora device 13
Mounted diagnostic cast 136
Mucosal insert 14

Nesbit prosthesis 14
Non-rigid connection (Table 3.2) 112
    hinge connection, joint 105

Obturator, velum 04
Occlusion 112
    occlusal scheme 138
    occlusal relationship 181
    centric relation 181
    centric occlusion 181
    long centric 180
    functionally generated 183
Palatal bar 26
Palatal strap 26
Partially edentulous state 01, 02
    effects of 02
    consequences of 02
    prosthesis selection for 02
    classification of (Kennedy's) ,06
    various classifications of (Table 1.1) 07
    terminology related to 11
Path of placement 14, 124
Percolation 95

Relief 25
Removable partial dentures 02
    rationale 04
    types of (extracoronal, intracoronal, tooth-borne,
        tooth-tissue borne) 05
    objectives 06
    rotational path 15
Resilient attachments 14
Resin bonded prosthesis 18
Rest and rest seat 15,50,51
    classification 50
    purpose 51
    support for 55
    types (occlusal, cingulum, incisal,
        quasi-cingulum, extended rest, onlay,
        embrssure rest) 51

Semiprecision attachment 15
Silanization 98
    of metal framework (Table 2.11) 98
Spoon denture 34
Sprue 15
Spruing of 168
    framework 168
    types of 171
    location of 171
Strees breaker prosthesis 18
Stress release clasp 68
    RPI, RPA, bar clasp, combination clasp 68
Sublingual bar 29
Support 151
Survey line 15
    Blatterfein's classification 75
Surveying 15,121
    surveyor, types of 122
        Ney122
        jelenko surveyor 122
        microanalyzer 122
        stress-o-graph 122
        Gimble stage table 123
        cast tilting for 127
Swing lock/hinged continuous bar 30

Tissue stops 45
Tooth alterations/modifications 140
Transitional prosthesis 03
Treatment denture 16

Undercut 16
U-shaped major connector 26

Wax pattern,166
Wrought 16